D0395216

Chicken Soup
for the Soul®

Say Hello to a Better Body!

Chicken Soup for the Soul: Say Hello to a Better Body!
Weight Loss and Fitness for Women Over 50
Dr. Suzanne Koven

Published by Chicken Soup for the Soul Health, an imprint of Chicken Soup for the Soul Publishing, LLC. www.chickensoup.com

Front cover and interior photo courtesy of iStockphoto.com/monkeybusinessimages
(© Catherine Yeulet). Back cover photo of Dr. Suzanne Koven courtesy of Pierre Chiha.

Cover and Interior Design & Layout by Pneuma Books, LLC
For more info on Pneuma Books, visit www.pneumabooks.com

Distributed to the booktrade by Simon & Schuster. SAN: 200-2442

Publisher's Cataloging-In-Publication Data
(Prepared by The Donohue Group, Inc.)

Koven, Suzanne.

   Chicken soup for the soul : say hello to a better body! : weight loss and fitness for women over 50 / Suzanne Koven.

   p. : ill. ; cm.

   Summary: A collection of stories on the topic of maintaining proper weight, exercising, and nutrition for women over 50, accompanied by medical advice and practical tips.

   ISBN: 978-1-935096-89-4

   1. Weight loss--Anecdotes. 2. Physical fitness for women--Anecdotes. 3. Older women--Health and hygiene--Anecdotes. 4. Weight loss--Popular works. 5. Physical fitness for women. 6. Older women--Health and hygiene.

PN6071.W45 K68 2012

810.2/02/356/1   2012931534

PRINTED IN THE UNITED STATES OF AMERICA
on acid∞free paper

21 20 19 18 17 16 15 14 13 12   01 02 03 04 05 06 07 08 09 10

Chicken Soup for the Soul

Say Hello to a Better Body!

Weight Loss and Fitness for Women Over 50

by **DR. SUZANNE KOVEN** of
HARVARD MEDICAL SCHOOL

CSS
Health

Chicken Soup for the Soul Publishing, LLC
Cos Cob, CT

Contents

Chapter 1
～ A Turning Point ～

Chapter 2
～ Taking Stock ～

Chapter 3
～ **Moving Forward** ～

Chapter 4
～ **Food for Thought** ～

Chapter 5
~ **The Long Run** ~

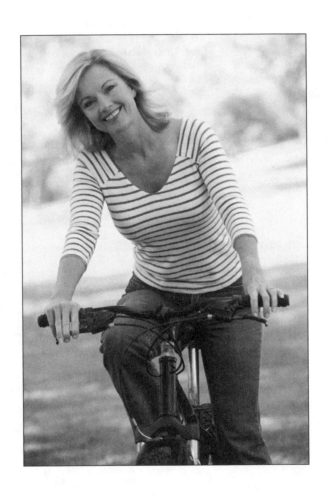

Chapter 1
A Turning Point

A Turning Point

Saying Hello

For over twenty years I've practiced medicine while my husband and I have raised our three kids. It's been a life filled with joys, challenges, disappointments, and pleasures. building a family and career, caring for aging parents and growing children, finding time for friendships, traveling, reading, gardening, volunteering, and, too rarely, just relaxing.

Whether you're married or single, a stay-at-home mom, re-tired, or work outside the home, live in the U.S., Canada, or else-where, I'm sure that as a woman over fifty you can recognize yourself in the picture I'm painting of a full and busy life.

As a woman over fifty reading this particular book, there's something else to which I think you will relate:

All during this time, amid these varied activities, one theme was constant for me, like a drum beating insistently in the back-ground: concern that my body was not as healthy as I wanted it to be.

By my thirties I'd moved beyond the years of fad dieting and obsession with a particular weight or jean size that had domi-nated my teens and twenties. But, as a young and then early middle-aged mother and doctor, I often ate too much, exercised too little, didn't get enough rest, and responded to the stress of increasing responsibilities at home and work by simply pushing myself harder.

Sometimes, for weeks or months at a time, I ate more healthfully, exercised more consistently, and made more time for relaxation. But these efforts always felt like, well, *efforts*: tedious and, inevitably, temporary fixes. And with each lapse back into old habits my confidence eroded still further that I'd ever be fit or make peace with my body.

When I turned fifty, yet a new variable entered this seemingly unsolvable equation: menopause. Practically overnight, I gained fifteen pounds, all in my waist—which had always been my trimmest area. Joints I didn't even know I had started to ache. Fatigue, which previously descended late each afternoon, began arriving earlier each day. My panicked attempt to reverse these changes with too-vigorous daily running resulted in a knee injury requiring surgery.

I wondered if I was destined to grow old and out of shape, having never really been *in* shape in the first place!

A turn in this discouraging state of affairs came from an unexpected source: my patients. Though, over the years, I'd tried just about all the usual (and some unusual) ways to lose weight and get fit that millions of other women have tried—too numerous to mention diets, exercise regimens, and even liposuction (it was new and they were offering steep discounts to student "guinea pigs")—it turned out that I had one avenue not available to the average woman: I acquired expertise in the medical management of obesity.

My colleagues began to refer patients who struggled with

their weight. I counseled these patients—mostly women—about how shedding excess weight could reduce their risk of heart disease, certain cancers, and a wide range of other conditions, including arthritis, depression, and sleep disorders. I helped them sort out the pros and cons of weight loss drugs and surgery. I reviewed their diets and exercise routines. And, in the process, I learned much that should have helped me get healthier, too.

But… it didn't.

After a while, I wondered if simply giving my patients information about weight loss and health was enough. After all, I'd learned lots of facts about nutrition and exercise, and I still struggled with my own weight and health habits. Let's face it: knowing how many fat grams are in a slice of pizza or how many calories are burned by jogging a mile (about 10 grams and 100 calories, respectively, in case you were wondering) is one thing, and passing up the pizza or saying yes to the jog are another. How could I best give my patients not only the information they needed, but also the tools to act on it—and not only for a few weeks, but for life?

You know the old proverb: "a problem shared is half solved?" I became convinced that rather than meeting with my patients one at a time, it would be beneficial to have them meet in groups so they could trade tips, and compare triumphs and struggles as they worked on losing weight and getting fit. I knew from what patients had confided to me over the years, and from my own experiences, that being overweight can feel very shameful and isolating. It's a huge relief to find out that you're not the only one who's ever hit the fast food drive-thru on your way home to dinner, hidden candy wrappers at the bottom of the garbage pail, or paid for membership in a health club you've never set foot in—and hugely motivating to hear that someone else managed to stop doing these things. Several studies support my impression that losing weight and exercising with a group or a buddy is more likely to lead to success.

So, with some of my colleagues, I started a group program for patients with diabetes, high cholesterol, and other conditions related to being overweight and inactive. Once a week we meet in a hospital conference room. Over yogurt, fresh fruit, and other healthy snacks, we talk about portion sizes and saturated fat, hamstring stretches and pulse rates, yoga and cardio. But the main thing we talk about is how to change our *minds*. For nearly all of us—and I include myself along with the patients here—the most challenging part of getting healthier is leaving behind decades of self-blame, perfectionism, and unrealistic expectations.

And the most powerful tool in changing our minds is hearing one another's stories, as you will in this book, which is like a weight loss and fitness support group you can hold in your hand.

As the weeks go by, new habits slowly replace old ones and participants begin to feel healthier, leaner, and calmer, mostly by adopting a few simple strategies. Here are just a few of those strategies—ones that I, as well as my patients, have found most useful:

- **Don't Follow Rules—Change Habits.** Instead of worrying about downing eight eight-ounce glasses of water a day, focus on keeping a water bottle on your desk and kitchen counter and drinking from it often.

Instead of counting saturated fat grams, start cooking with olive oil, low-fat dairy products, and leaner cuts of meat or vegetarian proteins. If the gym's not your thing, walk, take dancing lessons or plant a garden. Rules, as the saying goes, are made to be broken, but habits become part of your identity.

- **Make It Easy.** Join the pool or fitness club closer to your home or work. Stop buying chips and cookies "for the kids." (When *they're* over fifty, they'll thank you—obese children are much more likely to become obese adults.) Pack your lunch and gym bag the night before. The time most critical to the success of a weight loss or fitness plan are those few seconds when you're deciding: "Should I eat this, or that?" "Should I exercise, or skip it?" Make it as easy as possible to choose well by removing as many obstacles and temptations as you can.

- **Change Expectations.** Erase all the old "tapes" that have played in your head for years and have never helped you get fit. You know the ones I mean: *I need to lose two pounds every week. I need to get in shape by summer*, etc. I'll talk, at the end of this chapter, about other stale and unrealistic expectations that are best abandoned.

Meanwhile, you can also, gradually, change your

family's expectations about your behavior, about what kinds of foods you'll keep in the house, about the amount of time you need to take care of yourself, etc. You do this not with grand pronouncements such as "I'M ON A DIET!" or by asking your family to police you—how well has *that* ever worked?—but by the way you act, day in and day out. For example, my kids never call my cell phone, except for an emergency, during that regular hour when they know "Mom's working out."

- **Get Support.** Though groups such as the one I run, or those offered by commercial weight loss programs, can be very helpful, support comes in many other forms. A personal trainer, a walking buddy, or a yoga or healthy cooking class can all aid your fitness efforts. Any person or group who notices when you do or don't show up, applauds your progress, and cheers you on when you're feeling discouraged counts as support.

In this book you'll find lots of information about diet, exercise, stress management, injury prevention, and the countless health benefits of achieving and maintaining physical fitness.

But, even more importantly, you'll learn from the stories what the patients in my group have learned from one another: how to leave behind some of the psychological baggage that's been keeping you from incorporating this information into your daily life—your crazy, busy, wonderful life.

Not one woman who tells her story here achieved a "perfect" body, ate a 100% healthy diet, or exercised every single day without fail. Yet, I think you'll consider their stories successes. And the secret to these successes, as you'll see, lies in persistence, flexibility, and a sense of humor.

Be prepared to be inspired by a menopausal tango dancer, a middle-aged novice cook, a ninety-two-year-old yoga practitioner and many other women who decided, that over fifty is the perfect time to say hello to a better body.

I know I am.

Not Your Mother's Menopause

If you're a middle-aged woman, and you have the feeling that everything is changing—you're right!

First, there are the changes happening outside your body: your kids are likely leaving home or close to doing so; your parents need more of your attention, or pass away; your spouse, siblings, and friends start having health problems and/or think about retirement; and divorce, re-marriage, downsizing a home, and re-entering (or leaving) the workforce are common and dramatic transitions at this time of life.

Then, there are the changes happening inside your body: Usually beginning in a woman's early forties, the ovaries start decreasing their production of the hormone, estrogen, that makes pregnancy possible. This phase is called perimenopause. Eventually, the ovaries shut down altogether and menopause occurs. A woman is considered menopausal when she has stopped having menstrual periods for one year. The average age of menopause in the industrial world is fifty-one, though some women go through menopause as early as their late thirties and some as late as sixty.

The decrease in estrogen levels, as well as fluctuations in two other hormones — progesterone and testosterone — can cause women to experience many different symptoms and feelings. Some of the more familiar of these are: hot flashes, night sweats, weight gain, irritability, insomnia, vaginal dryness, and loss of sexual desire. Also common in perimenopause and menopause are increased intestinal gas, heart palpitations, depression, and difficulty concentrating.

Some women, it's important to mention, actually feel *better* during these years. Several surveys have identified women who have more energy, increased interest in and enjoyment of sex, and overall improved satisfaction with their lives around menopause. The hormonal changes that cause such distressing symptoms for some women may have the opposite effect on others. It's also possible that, at this time of life, many of us have more self-confidence, improved economic security, deeper relationships, fewer care-giving responsibilities, and more privacy and free time than when we were younger, and that these contribute to an improved sense of wellbeing.

For millennia, most women didn't have to worry about the changes — good or bad — that came with menopause: they didn't live long enough to experience them. A century ago, the average lifespan of the American woman was roughly fifty years. Now, women in the U.S. can expect, on average, to live nearly eighty years. This means we may live more than a third of our lives in menopause!

Over the last few decades, both society's and the medical profession's views about menopause have changed — and are still changing.

In 1966, a gynecologist named Robert Wilson wrote a widely popular book called *Feminine Forever*. Wilson argued that menopause was a disease, and that if women wanted to avoid becoming "dull and unattractive," they should take estrogen. The Women's Movement, not to mention the increased rates of uterine cancer among women who took estrogen, caused many to question the wisdom of Wilson's advice.

In the 1980s and 1990s, millions of menopausal and peri-menopausal women took a combination of estrogen and pro-gesterone. The most popular of the estrogens was synthesized from pregnant mare's urine, hence the name: Premarin. Adding progesterone (sometimes with estrogen in a combination pill called Prempro) protected women from the uterine cancer that estrogen can cause when taken alone. At the time it was thought that, in addition to alleviating hot flashes and other symptoms, these hormones prevented hip and other fractures caused by bone thinning (osteoporosis), cardiovascular disease, and Alzheimer's disease. When I first joined my medical prac-tice in 1990, it seemed that every woman I met over fifty was taking these hormones, whether she had menopausal symptoms or not.

Then, in 2002, a study from the Women's Health Initiative (WHI) showed that women who took estrogen and progesterone had an increased risk of breast cancer and, what's more, they were *more,* not less, likely to have heart attacks and strokes than women who hadn't taken the hormones. Overnight, millions of women stopped taking estrogen and progesterone. Now, doctors tend to prescribe estrogen and progesterone mostly for women who are having severe hot flashes, vaginal dryness, and other symptoms and, even then, not for more than a few years.

But the hormone story isn't over yet. The results of the WHI study are now being reconsidered because of two issues. The first is that the women in that study were, on average, in their sixties—usually several years past the onset of menopause. Also, the hormones used in that study, Premarin and similar medications, were synthetic. There are other hormones available, such as estradiol, called "bio-identical," that is, closer to those that occur naturally. Several studies are now underway to see if it's safe, and even beneficial, for younger women, those in their forties and fifties, to take these kinds of hormones.

Certainly, even before that information becomes available, you should discuss with your doctor whether hormone therapy is right for you. Women suffering from severe hot flashes, insomnia, irritability, and depression can often get fast and effective relief through hormone treatment. The distress that some women feel at menopause is real and can be disabling. I treated one of my patients with estrogen when, among other intolerable symptoms, she became so irritable she couldn't bear the sound of her husband's voice. (And she loved the guy. Really!) Cynthia Gorney, a journalist who described her decision to use estrogen in a 2010 *New York Times Magazine* article, wrote of those infamous perimenopausal mood swings: "I'm sorry, but only someone who has never experienced one could describe a day of 'I would stab everyone I know with a fork if only I could stop weeping long enough to get out of this car' as a 'mood swing.'"

But let's say you've decided that your symptoms aren't quite *that* bad, or you have a history of breast cancer, blood clots, or other conditions that make hormone treatment inadvisable, or you simply choose not to take hormones. Does that mean there's nothing you can do about some of the uncomfortable symptoms that can occur with menopause? No!

Research shows that women who exercise regularly have fewer hot flashes (or are less bothered by the hot flashes that they have). Limiting caffeine and alcohol also decreases the number and severity of hot flashes. Mood, metabolism, sleep, digestion, cognitive function, and even sexual function have all been shown to improve with exercise. A high fiber diet helps digestion. If you smoke, this is a perfect time to stop. Smoking accelerates the decline in estrogen levels and worsens perimenopausal symptoms—as well as increasing the risk for osteoporosis.

But alleviating the symptoms of perimenopause and menopause isn't the only reason to exercise, eat more healthfully, stop smoking, and adopt other healthy habits at this time of your life. Such habits can help make you stronger, more productive, and happier, for many more years than your mother and grandmother ever dreamed of.

New Seasons, New Reasons

There's no doubt that menopause makes it harder to lose weight and get fit. A slower metabolism, decrease in muscle mass, stiff and sore joints, increased sugar cravings, and fatigue from disrupted sleep all make getting in shape more challenging as we get older. However, middle-aged women do have some advantages:

For one thing, we have more confidence than when we were younger. We're less likely to feel self-conscious about making a special order in a restaurant or showing up at the gym without the coolest outfit than we might been have years ago.

We're older and wiser. We know from experience that thirty days don't, actually, lead to thinner thighs and that the stuff they advertise on late night TV and in the backs of magazines doesn't melt pounds away while you sleep.

We're also often more motivated than we were in the past. The reasons to get fit are more meaningful to us. The stakes seem higher. How important is fitting into a particular pair of shorts compared with living to see your grandchildren grow up? How satisfying does a certain number on the scale seem next to having the energy to pursue that second career? Continue living independently? Prevent cancer?

Time after time I've seen women who've tried for years to lose weight finally succeed when they have a goal that really means something to them. An example is Suzanne Ruff, whose story, "Tending My Rose Garden," you'll read here. She was so upset about being heavy that she decided to stop shopping for clothes altogether. But it wasn't until her sister became desperately ill and needed a healthy kidney donor that Suzanne found the will to get in shape. Mary Elizabeth Laufer, the author of "The Whistle that Woke Me Up," had packed away her too-small clothes and, with them, all hope of ever losing weight, until her doctor told her she had high blood pressure.

If you've not yet found powerful motivation for adopting a healthier lifestyle, here are some recent research findings worth thinking about:

- Post-menopausal women who walk 30 minutes per day lower their risk for breast cancer by 20%. Obese women in this age group are 30-50% more likely than thinner women to develop breast cancer.

- Women who replace animal fats with vegetable oils in their diets cut their risk of heart attack in half.

- Women who are chronically stressed, depressed, angry, or socially isolated are more likely to die of heart disease. Older women who have a strong network of friends are much less likely to die of heart disease than those with weaker social support.

- Exercising, quitting smoking, and getting diabetes and high blood pressure under control markedly reduce a middle-aged woman's chances of ending up in a nursing home later in life.

- Exercise boosts brain power. Regular workouts improve intellectual capacity, creativity, and even empathy. The brain scans of adults who exercise actually demonstrate growth of gray matter. Exercisers are less likely to develop dementia, and exercise can slow the progression of memory loss in people who already have it.

- Regular weight-bearing exercise and a diet rich in calcium and vitamin D can help prevent osteoporosis. One in two women will break a bone at some point because of osteoporosis. An older woman who breaks her hip has a 25% chance of dying within a year.

- It's never too late to reap the health benefits of exercise. Even women in their nineties can sometimes stop using their canes after following a simple strength training routine.

The bottom line? Small changes every day—trading mayonnaise for olive oil in salad dressing, meeting a friend for a walk rather than watching TV alone, lifting a 3-pound weight instead of a cigarette, can, when added up, drastically improve your quality of life in the years to come—and may even be the difference between life and death.

Sounds like a pretty good deal, doesn't it?

Letting Go, Holding On

So you've decided to embark on a weight loss and fitness program and you're excited about it, but you're a bit apprehensive, too. After all, you've tried to get in shape so many times before. Your past is littered with abandoned treadmills, warped aerobics videos, and countless food journals, calorie counters, and packets of artificial sweetener. And you're in good company. It's estimated that on any given day, half of all American girls and women are trying to lose weight. One study from the U.K. estimated that, on average, British women spend thirty-one years of their lives on diets.

The bad news is that, by the time you're in your fifties, you've likely accrued a long history of repeated failure with regard to weight loss and fitness and, understandably, your confidence that you'll ever succeed is shaky.

The good news is, that at this time of life, you may finally be ready to let go of some of the self-defeating attitudes that have hampered your efforts.

I once wrote a blog for *Psychology Today* in which I coined the term "the un-nesting Instinct." I was referring to the urge that many women feel, at menopause, to de-clutter their lives, both physically and emotionally. This urge—the opposite of the drive to "feather the nest" that made many of us fill linen closets and refrigerators when we were pregnant—can take several forms: We may, finally, feel moved to empty the garage, give away our kids' old books and toys, end relationships that haven't felt nourishing, or mend fences with people with whom we've been in conflict.

This desire to "clean house" can be put to good use in your weight loss and fitness efforts. Those mental "tapes" to which I referred earlier have not really helped you get in shape, have they? Maybe it's time to pack them up, along with those wooden tennis rackets and dusty Sesame Street puppets, and make room for some new ideas.

Here are some "oldies but baddies"—untrue and unhelpful things you've probably been telling yourself for far too long:

- *I have no willpower, no self-discipline.* Really? Aren't you the same woman who raised those kids? Showed up for work every day? Cared for all those sick friends and relatives? My own experience counseling women who struggle with their weight is that they are unusually self-disciplined, and that, in fact, often food is the only aspect of their lives in which they allow themselves to lose control. Furthermore, recent research in behavioral psychology suggests that we may be thinking of willpower the wrong way: it's not something you're born with—like blue eyes or red hair—it's more like a muscle you strengthen with repeated use.

- *I'm good for a while, but then I always cheat.* What's with the moral self-judgment? The last time I looked, "Thou shalt not eat Doritos straight from the bag" is not one of the Ten Commandments. Your diet and exercise habits do not make you a bad (or good)

person. Believing that they do causes a lot of unnec-
essary stress—which drives many of us to overeat!

- *I've blown it for today, so I guess I'll just skip my
  workout and eat even more.* As my patient, Tina, put
  it, this makes about as much sense as getting a flat
  tire, and then deliberately puncturing the other three.
  Lose the all-or-nothing, black-and-white thinking.

- *I'll get in shape when work slows down, in time for
  my daughter's wedding, starting Monday morning...*
  Somehow, the "right time" never comes, or it *does*
  come, and then the next roadblock or artificial dead-
  line looms. Besides, being busy and stressed out is a
  good reason to take *better*, not worse, care of yourself. Mary, a participant in my group, was tempted to
  drop her new walking program when her daughter's
  cancer relapsed. Then she realized that a daily walk
  would increase her ability to cope with her daughter's illness.

The "right time" is now. This very minute. And the next. And
the next...

As you're questioning some old, ineffective approaches, take
some time to review ways of thinking and behaving that have
worked for you. Reflect on something you're proud of having
accomplished: mastering a skill such as quilting or playing the

piano; tackling a home renovation or major project at work; planning a special vacation, or your retirement. How did you do it? Did you seek the guidance of experts? Then maybe you'd find a class, personal trainer or dietician helpful as you try to get in shape. Or perhaps you enjoyed working on your own, at your own pace? Then maybe formal instruction is not for you. If you have a creative streak, then a dance class, journal writing, or experimenting with new recipes could be part of your weight loss strategy. A numbers person? You might have fun with one of the many free online sites and smart phone apps available for tracking diet and exercise.

As much as possible, play to your strengths rather than struggling against your challenges. To borrow a phrase from Boston-based health coach Margaret Moore, you want your fitness plan to feel "less like a wrestling match and more like a dance."

Albert Einstein once wrote: "We cannot solve our problems with the same thinking we used when we created them." At mid-life, many of us may feel that an overweight and unhealthy body is a "problem" we can never overcome. But I've known many women — and this book is filled with the stories of women — who did just that. And, as Einstein implied, changing our thinking is the first, and perhaps most important, step.

A Better Kind of
Hot Flash

N o one should have to go through menopause and divorce at the same time. That's just what I did, though. A hot flash came as I was signing the papers, and I knew this time it wasn't just anger or disappointment. My heart raced, and my forehead perspired so heavily that drops of sweat fell on the documents.

"My ex better not think those are tears," I joked to the lawyer before I fled to the washroom. "Maybe we should clarify that in the margins and initial it."

"Oh God," I moaned into the sink, "why is this happening to me?" I turned from my reflection, but not before seeing myself with uncomfortable clarity—a stiffly hunched middle-aged woman. While the marriage was breaking up, I stopped taking care of myself. I was too depressed to exercise, and I ate my way out of my feelings. Now, here I was, fifty-two years old, single, and forty pounds overweight. I locked myself into a toilet stall and cried.

When the tears passed, I washed my face and composed myself. I returned to the office, paid my fees and left. My lawyer's office is next to the Methodist church, and on a whim, I walked into the church to pray. I spent some time on my knees but nothing happened. Feeling foolish, I walked out sheepishly into the lobby. A flyer on the bulletin board caught my eye. Smiling, I wrote down the phone number. As always, God has a funny way of answering prayers, in this case with the tango.

At my first class, I learned about the practice embrace. You put your hands on a stranger's shoulders, and he puts his hands on yours. There is space between you, but you're connected, hearts open, chests facing one another. Within the first eight steps, I was hooked.

"Tango opens the heart," the instructor told us. "And it gives you great legs," joked Patricia, a grandmother and classmate who had been dancing for more than four years.

I had noticed that right away. Not one of the women was under the age of fifty, but they all had legs even Betty Grable would have envied. Their hair was gray but their waists were lithe, their arms toned, their posture graceful, their legs sculpted and strong, and most importantly, they had a glow. They didn't look young, but they looked beautiful, alive.

"Tango is just walking," the instructor said, "but walking in the most graceful, aware attitude possible. Feel your partner. Feel the music. Feel yourself. Never lose contact with the floor."

This was advice I could follow—on the dance floor and off it. For the first six months I tangoed twice a week. Then three times. I began to attend milongas (dance gatherings for tangueros), first in my city, then around the state. And as the dance strengthened and refined my body, it also changed my attitude. When a setback came I remained open. When I felt self-pity or resentment, I stayed in contact with the ground. When I felt sad or lost, I connected with the people around me.

I let myself receive their cues—their love, their warmth—just as I learned to listen to the wordless cues of a dance partner. In tango I learned to trust the strangers who held me in their arms; they became, over time, friends. I trusted the lead; I trusted the music; I trusted myself.

The exercise seemed like a fringe benefit at first. But then people started saying things. "Wow, what's different about you? Have you lost weight?"

I had lost weight around my hips, off my thighs, and best of all, I'd lost the weight that was on my heart. For the first time in years I moved my body in celebration. This was more than exercise!

For the first six months, I learned to dance in that open practice embrace. But finally, at a milonga in the upstairs rec room of the church where I'd first found the flyer, my partner popped the question.

"Now," he said, "are you ready for the close embrace?" He opened his arms and pulled me near. I blushed like a teenager. For a moment all my doubts flooded back. Was I ready? Then the music thumped. My partner led me into a series of backward ochos. My face was burning, but my body knew the steps. I relaxed. He pulled me closer until we were dancing cheek to cheek.

Dancing cheek to cheek. I'd heard the song, seen it in movies, but never experienced it myself. Not when I was young and pretty. Not until I was past fifty and in the best shape, mentally and physically, of my life. Better late than never. Believe me, it was worth the wait.

— Helen Reeves —

Tending My Rose Garden

The zipper wouldn't budge. I inhaled deeply, sucked in my gut and buttoned the top button on the slacks. Then I yanked the zipper closed and exhaled. I gazed at myself in the dressing room mirror.

I looked like a stuffed sausage!

"Here you go!" a sickeningly cheerful voice chirped on the other side of the dressing room door.

Grimacing, I pulled open the door and reached for the clothes the saleswoman handed me. "I brought you a dress to try, too!" Seeing my look of frustration, she cooed, "The larger sizes will probably fit, dear. I'm sure one of them will work!"

"I just had a baby, okay?" I snarled and slammed the door on her astonished face. Well, maybe not just... my youngest child was twenty-five years old!

Okay, so I lied. I have children—grown children—but this changing body of mine feels like it is going through the up-heaval of pregnancy.

It's called menopause (or mean-o-pause as my husband whispers to our family when he thinks I don't hear him). My body was betraying me, I thought, as I looked in the mirror. I'd gone up two sizes in the last couple of years. Could that really be me in the mirror? I looked like my grandmother when

I tried that dress! Why did they have such hideous lighting in these dressing rooms?

My belly protruded, my skin sagged, and my double chins were highlighted in the three-way mirror. Tears stung my eyes as I tried on the next item.

I was done shopping. I left without a purchase and went home dejected. My fiftieth birthday was approaching and a party was planned. I realized I had avoided shopping because I didn't want to subject myself to the exact kind of humiliation I had just experienced.

"I'll wear something I already have to the party!" I wailed to my sister, JoAnn. "You just wait! You'll be in the same boat next year. Fifty is terrifying!" My sister was thirteen months and thirteen days younger.

I continued my rant, "When I tend my rose garden, I've often thought women are like roses. When we hit puberty, we are like the bud on a rose. When that bud unfurls, it's magical. Slowly, like a girl growing into womanhood, the rosebud transforms into a full and beautiful rose. The flower brightens the garden and draws your eye. Eventually, a petal drifts down to the ground, and then another petal, the way women start to lose their looks as they age. When all the petals fall off—well, you know."

"Aah, stop your bellyaching!" my sister chided me. "You'll probably wear your usual black and white!"

The following year came. When JoAnn turned fifty years old, she looked like a skeleton. Family and friends whispered about her shocking appearance. She brushed us off, saying it had been a bad year. Our mother had died suddenly and JoAnn's husband lost his job that year. JoAnn said she was stressed, plus she was working extra hours to earn more money.

At a holiday gathering just before Christmas, I watched her toy with her food. I half-heartedly joked, "It's not fair. I'm short and you're tall. I get fat and you get skinnier." Deep down, though, I was very concerned.

A few days later, my other sister, Janice, telephoned me. "JoAnn collapsed and is in the hospital. She's in critical condition. I'll call you when they know what's wrong."

Terrified, I hung up the telephone. When Janice called me back, she told me JoAnn had "the disease." In our family, that meant polycystic kidney disease (PKD). Our mother had PKD and Janice has PKD and now JoAnn had it, too. It is a genetic disease that causes many cysts to grow and cover the kidneys, causing them to fail. There is no cure. The only treatment is dialysis—a machine that cleanses your blood the way your kidneys do—or transplantation.

I knew "the disease" well. Many of the people I loved most battled it. Eight family members lost their lives to PKD including our mother and grandmother, aunts and uncles. One of our cousins died while waiting for a kidney transplant.

I knew what JoAnn's life would be like because our mother had spent almost ten years of her life on dialysis. I knew there are not enough organ donors. When I finally talked to JoAnn, I blurted, "JoAnn, I will give you one of my kidneys."

Despite her own situation, JoAnn was concerned for me.

She didn't take my offer seriously. One, she wanted me to be sure I didn't have the disease. Two, she didn't think I'd have the courage to give her a kidney. She knew I was terrified of hospitals, needles and illness.

I didn't have the disease. I did give her one of my kidneys.

Twelve weeks before the surgery, I hired a personal trainer and got myself in the best shape I could before surgery. On the morning of the transplant, raw emotion made her voice raspy when JoAnn whispered, "I didn't think you'd be here! You can change your mind, you know!" She had told me that many times during the months before the surgery.

"I didn't think I'd be here either, but I'm not changing my mind," I told her as I went off to surgery.

The surgery was a success; we are both well. Seven years later, JoAnn lives a normal life, although she will always have the disease and need medication.

I had forgotten to closely observe the roses in my garden. After a rosebud blossoms into a flower and loses its petals, a rose hip appears on the cane where the rosebud began. Rose hips are lovely, useful and another part of the rose's beauty. Rose hips turn a stunning red color in autumn. I'm in the rose hip cycle of life.

A body blessed without disease humbled me. It responds well to good nutrition, exercise and a balanced life. My body is a glorious, magical, fabulous wonder. Despite its bulges, sagging parts, varicose veins, calluses, wrinkles, stretch marks and scars, it performs the magic we call life each day. Life!

Giving one of my body parts to keep that magic alive in

my sister fills me with gratitude and awe. My body is a temple I give thanks for each day.

~ Suzanne F. Ruff ~

Getting
the Picture

My entire adult life I've thought, "Once this project is complete I will have some rest. When this event is over things will calm down. As soon as this holiday passes, I'll lose weight." Guess what I finally learned? There are always new projects. Things never calm down. And the holidays keep coming.

I opened the mailbox and found a card from my sister-in-law with a picture of my mom, my sister and me taken at our family's Christmas get-together. She included a small note that said, "I hope you like the picture." Well,.. I didn't. It wasn't a conscious decision then, but that picture started me on my weight loss journey.

I am 4'10" with a small frame. At my heaviest, I wore a size 1X and topped the scale at a whopping 206 pounds with a body mass index of 43. It was definitely time to quit waiting and make some important changes. After a couple of months of thoughtful research, I signed up for a medically supervised weight loss program, determined to succeed with a healthy plan I could learn from, live with, and incorporate into a permanent lifestyle.

The first week of the plan was challenging but not unbearable. The second week seemed easier and I moved smoothly but a bit tentatively into the third week. Fortunately at this strategic point, a series of events happened that increased my momentum and confirmed I was in the right program at the right time.

As I walked on the treadmill listening to my radio, I heard a San Diego pastor discussing his own challenge with being overweight and living an unhealthy lifestyle. Pastor Jim talked about his motivation and described the medically supervised program that helped him lose ninety pounds. He addressed each step, the classes and the phases he went through. Though he didn't identify the program, it sounded incredibly familiar. The following Monday when I checked in for my weight appointment there was an article hanging next to the reception window—Pastor Jim's personal testimony on his success in our weight management program.

A week later I listened to nutritionist and speaker David Meinz. His healthy approach to eating was peppered with humor and a common sense attitude toward healthy lifestyle choices. I was so impressed that I bought his book and the CD of the program. However, it was a third incident that confirmed how my weight gain had undermined my health, and why I had no choice but to succeed.

An irritating, itchy red blotch, the size of a nickel, appeared directly above my right cheekbone. As the itching worsened, it grew larger. I went to my doctor, who prescribed an antifungal cream. I battled the spot for a couple of weeks until one morning I woke up with new spots on my face. By the time I left for work I had welts on one of my hands. I pulled up to the office ten minutes later, and my lips were covered, inside and out, with welts. No doubt I was having an allergic reaction. My doctor took one look at me, glanced quickly through my chart and said, "This definitely isn't a fungus. It's an allergic reaction to your blood pressure medication."

This was not the first time I had encountered a challenge with my medications. Or even the second. Here I was again, trying to find a new medication that I wasn't allergic to and that my insurance would cover.

I stomped out of the doctor's office muttering under my breath and headed towards the pharmacy with a new prescription... again. I got into my car, slammed the door, and buckled my seatbelt. As I sat there fuming I had an epiphany. I had been angry with the doctor, the pharmacy, and the insurance company. I blamed them all—for choosing wrong medications, for constantly changing the drugs they covered, and for the high cost of the prescriptions. Suddenly that blame traveled full circle and rested squarely where it belonged. All those times I was angry, it wasn't their fault... it was mine. The truth is that it's possible that if my weight hadn't spiraled out of control, I wouldn't have needed those medications. I was the problem, not the drugs.

I surprised myself throughout the weight loss portion of the program by sticking to it. I stayed within the allowed food choices, diligently did everything that was expected and successfully transitioned into maintaining my weight. For me, that was the scary part. My fears centered on the maintenance phase when my choices would broaden.

One of the most interesting phenomena I observed in my journey is how many people are unhappy with their weight and their health, yet unwilling to change their attitudes and behaviors. I've seen many people struggle with their weight loss while I have been on my program. They face some of the same issues of control and emotional challenges that I have. They consistently eat food not on their plan. Each week, as they step on the scale, they make another excuse for not losing weight. They become frustrated because they aren't moving toward their goal. Why? Because they haven't learned that if we want our lives to change, we must change.

No one can nag, embarrass, bully, trick or manipulate you into losing weight. For me it took that nudge from my prescription medicine allergy, the deciding moment when I finally understood and accepted the responsibility to live a healthier life. Most of us know that we need to make that decision but we aren't ready. The first step to a healthier life is to recognize the need for change. The next is to weigh the options and choose a reasonable, reliable, and workable health plan and goal for weight loss and maintenance that will work for us. Then we have to make a commitment to do what is necessary to accomplish that goal.

Nine months into the program I weighed 104 pounds with a BMI of 22 and wore a size two. Six years later I still firmly believe that when we want something to change in our lives permanently, we must make permanent changes. It took me quite a while to see things clearly and figure that out, but with a little nudge and a lot of determination, I've finally got the picture.

— Valerie J. Frost —

The Whistle that Woke Me Up

Whn I moved across the country because of my husband's new job, I left behind sunny Orlando, Florida for overcast Portland, Oregon. I no longer spent my free time swimming and playing tennis. Instead, I sat in front of the computer e-mailing old friends.

Soon my face looked rounder and my pants felt tight. I searched my closet for something to wear and found that half my clothes didn't fit me anymore. When did I get fat?

The extra weight didn't go away, and I slowly accepted it as an inevitable part of growing older. After all, my siblings and friends had also gained weight as they aged. I boxed up the clothes I'd outgrown and took them to Goodwill. It was time to give up the fantasy of ever fitting into them again.

The next time I went for a physical, the doctor pointed out that my blood pressure was high. And when he saw my weight, he whistled. Whistled! I felt like crying. It wasn't my fault! Wasn't gaining weight just a normal part of midlife?

"Join a gym," the doctor said.

A gym? Me? It conjured up bad memories of high school. "I can't afford it," I said.

"Then walk."

"But it rains every day!" I protested.

"You won't melt."

The truth is I was afraid of getting struck by lightning. But this rude doctor would probably have laughed at me if I told him that.

When my blood work came back, there was more bad news. My LDL was too high and my HDL was too low. My blood sugar was abnormal, too. I had to return to take a glucose fasting test, and the diagnosis came back pre-diabetes.

Was I going to end up like my parents, with prescription bottles lined up on the counter, and several pills a day to keep track of for the rest of my life?

Our local hospital had a health education center that offered free courses on staying healthy. In desperation, I signed up for one. I'd spent most of my adult life caring for my kids. Maybe it was time to start taking care of myself.

I barraged the instructor with questions. How could I lower my blood pressure? Raise my HDL? Stabilize my blood sugar? I listened to a lot of information about cutting down on salt and eating a plant-based diet. But for every medical problem I had, one remedy kept getting mentioned. Exercise! Exercise! Exercise!

My doctor was right. I needed to walk. I quickly got over my fear of lightning when I realized Portland's skies rarely produced it, unlike the skies in Orlando, which was the lightning capital of the United States. When it rained here, I could carry an umbrella and not feel as if I were holding a miniature lightning rod.

Miles of sidewalks connected my subdivision. I went outside first thing in the morning, before I could invent excuses not to, and just started walking.

"Out for a stroll?" my neighbor asked me.

"A power walk!" I answered. After a few blocks I broke out in a sweat, and then came home and showered.

Every day I went a little farther. I bought a pocket calendar and recorded how long I walked: twenty minutes, twenty-five, thirty. I also stood on the scale every day and then wrote down my weight. Slowly it began to go down.

Gradually I worked up to walking forty-five minutes a day. One morning I saw a woman walking ahead of me and struck up a conversation with her. Her name was Claudette and she lived on the next block. I started phoning her before I went out to ask if she wanted to walk with me. Soon I just met her at her house at eight every morning and we walked together. Walking went faster when we talked. We chatted about our kids and our husbands, about religion and politics. I not only had a walking partner, I had a friend!

Claudette and I were like mailmen. Every day, come rain, sleet or snow, we walked our route. People would smile and wave at us. They probably thought we were crazy. Because I was used to warm Florida winters, I bundled up in a heavy jacket, knit hat, corduroys, thick socks and a scarf over my face. Claudette usually donned just a hoodie. We both wore out several pairs of sneakers.

Walking became a priority. If anything came up that might prevent me from doing it, I always worked around it. I would go out to walk earlier, or walk afterward. If Claudette couldn't go for some reason, I went anyway. Seven days a week.

Ice was the only thing that still scared me. I didn't want to slip and fall and break my bones! On really cold mornings the sidewalks in the shade glazed over. Claudette and I had some close calls where we almost fell but caught each other in the nick of time. So I bought a stepper at a garage sale that I could use at home on icy mornings. I also had a *Pilates for Dummies* tape for backup.

My wedding ring began to slip off. My face looked thinner and my thighs firmer. I would have fit into all the clothes I'd given away! And I felt great. One wonderful benefit of exercise is that it alleviates depression. I didn't even know that I'd been depressed until I began to feel better.

The next time I went to my doctor, I couldn't wait for him to ask me how I'd lost twenty pounds. I was ready to tell him how his whistle had woken me up, and how since then I'd dedicated myself to walking. But to my surprise, he didn't say a word about my weight. He frowned when he looked at my chart and afterward handed me a slip of paper to get blood work.

It was only when I went to the lab for my blood work that I realized my weight loss had made an impact on him.

"The results of your thyroid test should be back in a couple of days," the nurse said.

My thyroid test? And then it hit me. The doctor attributed my weight loss to an out-of-kilter thyroid! As if I couldn't have lost this much weight on my own!

Oh, well. It didn't matter what the doctor thought. My

thyroid test came back normal. My LDL was down now, and my HDL was up. My blood sugar was no longer in the pre-diabetic range. I had done it all myself, simply by putting one foot in front of the other.

— Mary Elizabeth Laufer —

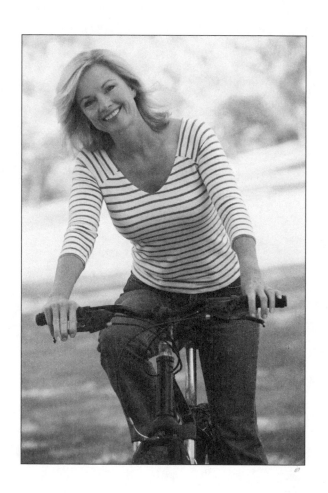

Chapter 2
Taking Stock

Taking Stock

You Are HERE

You know those maps in shopping malls and on hiking trails? They always include a circle labeled "You are HERE." Similarly, when you turn on the GPS in your car, it identifies your current location before calculating a route. The truth is, you can't get where you want to go if you don't know where you are.

The very first step in your journey to lose weight and get fit isn't buying new cookbooks or signing up with a personal trainer. Before taking actions such as these, you need to do a little mental preparation. When I say this to the participants in my cardiovascular prevention group, they look at me like I've gone off the deep end. "What is there to think about?" they groan. "We've been thinking about losing weight and living a healthier lifestyle for years!" Perhaps you would say the same.

And yet, when I ask my patients to explain *why* they want to lose weight, or even to tell me whether they feel ready to make changes in their lives, they realize that despite years of on and off dieting and exercising, they've never really thought about these two very basic questions. Would you say the same?

On a piece of paper, copy these two questions and write down your answers:

1. Why do I want to lose weight and get fit? (In other words, why is it meaningful to me?)

2. How ready am I to make the permanent changes in my behavior necessary to meet theses goals? Am I:
   a. Not even thinking about it.
   b. Thinking about it, but not ready to act.
   c. Making preparations to act (e.g., joined a gym, made an appointment with a dietician, etc.)
   d. Already starting to make changes.
   e. Accustomed to changes, which are a regular part of my life.

It's preferable to write out the answers with pen and paper, in your own handwriting, as if signing a contract—which, in a sense, it is: a contract with yourself.

The answer to question #1 is your motivation. It may change, over time, but it is crucial to articulate it as specifically and as honestly as you can. Are you adopting new habits so that you can: Have enough energy to start a new business? Live to see your grandchildren grow up? Avoid the chronic diseases that plagued your parents? Simply to feel better than you do right now? The answer that is truest for you, personally, is your most powerful tool in losing weight and getting fit—but you must fully acknowledge and own it.

Question # 2, adapted from the "Stages of Change" devised by psychologist James Prochaska, gives you some important information as well. I'm assuming that if you are reading this book, you are not at "a," and probably not at "e," either (though even women who have already made lifestyle changes may be looking for new challenges). Prochaska's insight was that these stages are like building blocks, and you can't skip over one to rush to the next. For example, if you're browsing through these pages, daydreaming about a healthier life, it likely won't be effective to wake up tomorrow morning and, having done no preparation whatsoever, just decide to start eating better and exercising. And, come to think of it… how often have you tried to do just that, with disappointing results?

So now that you've written down your motivation for losing weight and getting fit, and assessed your readiness to work on those goals, it's time to take a clear-eyed look at just how much excess weight you currently carry, as well as your level of fitness.

Let's start with your weight. If you've been dieting on and off for many years, you likely have a "magic number," a weight that you think is "ideal." But it's very possible that this number is unnecessarily low and that you need to lose less weight than you think in order to significantly improve your health.

Doctors and medical researchers now use a measurement called "body-mass index" (BMI) to determine whether people are at a healthy weight. You can calculate your BMI manually by plugging your height and weight into a mathematical equation (see below) — but it's easier to use one of the many online calculators or a chart such as the one here.

$$BMI = \left\{ \frac{\text{WEIGHT (pounds)}}{\text{HEIGHT (inches)}^2} \right\} \times 703$$

TABLE 1 What's your body mass index?													
Height	Weight in pounds												
4'10"	91	96	100	105	110	115	119	124	129	134	138	143	167	191
4'11"	94	99	104	109	114	119	124	128	133	138	143	148	173	198
5'0"	97	102	107	112	118	123	128	133	138	143	148	153	179	204
5'1"	100	106	111	116	122	127	132	137	143	148	153	158	185	211
5'2"	104	109	115	120	126	131	136	142	147	153	158	164	191	218
5'3"	107	113	118	124	130	135	141	146	152	158	163	169	197	225
5'4"	110	116	122	128	134	140	145	151	157	163	169	174	204	232
5'5"	114	120	126	132	138	144	150	156	162	168	174	180	210	240
5'6"	118	124	130	136	142	148	155	161	167	173	179	186	216	247
5'7"	121	127	134	140	146	153	159	166	172	178	185	191	223	255
5'8"	125	131	138	144	151	158	164	171	177	184	190	197	230	262
5'9"	128	135	142	149	155	162	169	176	182	189	196	203	236	270
5'10"	132	139	146	153	160	167	174	181	188	195	202	207	243	278
5'11"	136	143	150	157	165	172	179	186	193	200	208	215	250	286
6'0"	140	147	154	162	169	177	184	191	199	206	213	221	258	294
6'1"	144	151	159	166	174	182	189	197	204	212	219	227	265	302
6'2"	148	155	163	171	179	186	194	202	210	218	225	233	272	311
6'3"	152	160	168	176	184	192	200	208	216	224	232	240	279	319
6'4"	156	164	172	180	189	197	205	213	221	230	238	246	287	328
BMI	19	20	21	22	23	24	25	26	27	28	29	30	35	40
	NORMAL						OVERWEIGHT					OBESE		

*From a Harvard Health Publications Special Health Report: *Diabetes: a plan for living.*

BMI gives a rough estimate of total body fat. It's not accurate in people who have large muscles (which are heavy, but not made of fat) and, over the past few years, the criteria for "normal," "overweight," and "obese" have been revised a bit. But knowing your BMI still gives you a pretty good idea of whether you need to lose weight and how much.

Weigh yourself and have your height measured (after menopause, thinning of the bones in your spine may have caused you to lose an inch or two), and then find your BMI on this chart. If you are in the "obese" range, what is the least amount of weight you'd need to lose to get into the "over-weight" range? And if you are "overweight," what's the least amount of weight you need to lose to get to "normal? Those are good goals for now.

The most important, and most encouraging, thing to know about BMI is that the heavier you are, the less weight loss it takes to make a big impact on your health. Take a look at this graph. It shows how the risk of dying prematurely (from heart disease, stroke, diabetes, and other conditions) rises with increasing body weight:

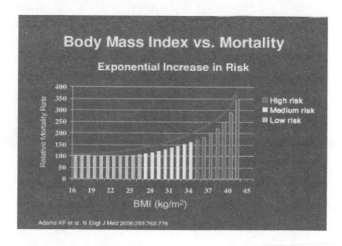

Depending on how you view it, this could be a really scary graph, since it shows that going from a BMI of 34 to a BMI of 40 (that's a gain of just 30 pounds for a 5'4" woman) doubles your likelihood of dying early. I like to think of it a different way: If you're a 5'4" woman who weighs 230 pounds, you can cut your risk of dying prematurely in half simply by getting to 200 pounds! That may not be your final goal—optimally, you should try to get into the normal range—but you can accomplish quite a lot with a more modest weight loss.

It may take some psychological adjustment to set a weight goal that's much higher than your old "magic number." Many of us have long carried around a distorted view of what we "should" weigh. I realized this recently when a friend and I were leafing through pictures of ourselves at her wedding thirty years ago. "Look how thin we were," we both said, "When we thought we were fat!"

Beyond the Scale

Weight (or BMI) isn't the only measure of fitness. If you're overweight and you work out regularly, you may be more fit than your skinny friend who never lifts anything heavier than her cell phone. And even two women who have the same BMI may have different degrees of health risk from their excess pounds.

People who accumulate extra weight in their waists ("apples") have a greater risk of heart disease than people who carry extra weight in their hips ("pears"). Extra weight around the midsection, which sometimes first appears during menopause, can be a sign of the internal or "visceral" fat you've heard can cause heart disease, inflammation, and other health problems. It's a common misconception that excess belly fat is impossible to shed after menopause, but that's not true, as April Knight, author of "Reunion," discovered.

A quick way to determine if you're an "apple" is to measure your waist across the navel. If it's 35 inches or greater (40 inches, for men), you likely fit the riskier "apple" profile. If, in addition to having extra weight in your midsection, you also have high blood pressure, and certain abnormal blood tests (see below) you may have what's called "metabolic syndrome." This syndrome, affecting nearly a quarter of all American women, greatly increases your risk of developing heart disease and diabetes. It's important to know if you have metabolic syndrome. If you do, getting active and eating healthier are all the more crucial. Metabolic syndrome *can* be reversed

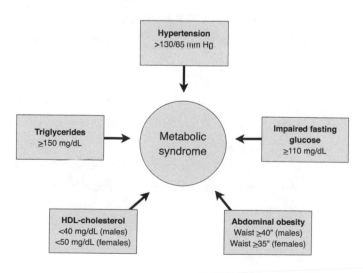

In addition to knowing your weight, BMI, and waist size, it's helpful to be aware of some other measures of fitness. Cardiovascular (or aerobic) endurance, strength, flexibility, and balance all contribute to your health and wellbeing. After all, besides achieving a healthy weight, you also want to be able to avoid falls, run for a bus, and say "No thanks, I've got it!" when a younger person offers to hoist your suitcase into the overhead bin. The website www.adultfitnesstest.org, sponsored by the President's Council on Physical Fitness and Sports, provides simple tests of various types of fitness. Repeat these tests periodically to see how far you've progressed. If you are now completely inactive, though, do not undertake tests such as brisk walking or running without first consulting your doctor.

A Health Inventory

I've seen smart women do some pretty dumb things in order to lose weight: starvation diets, extreme exercise routines, and over the counter or even illegal appetite suppressants. These unhealthy strategies never work in the long run, partly because they make you feel so awful. Who can stick to a plan that makes you hungry, achy, or jittery? It works much better—and makes much more sense, especially when you're over fifty—to think of losing weight as part of an overall health improvement plan: one you're motivated to stay with because, in addition to preventing illness, it makes you feel good.

So, as you're taking stock of your weight and fitness, take a few minutes to look at the big picture of your health. Here are some questions you might ask yourself about your general medical care:

- Have I had a check up with my doctor in the last year? Am I up to date on all recommended cancer screening tests (mammograms, Pap smears, etc.) and immunizations?
- Have I had a bone density test to screen for osteoporosis (bone thinning)?
- Have I reviewed all my medications, including over-the-counter drugs and supplements, with my doctor? Am I taking anything, such as certain hormones and psychiatric medications, that causes weight gain? (Do NOT stop any medication without first consulting your doctor.)
- Am I due for a dental or eye exam? The condition of your teeth and gums can affect your heart and overall health, and poor vision can cause falls and derail an exercise program.

And, just as important to your health as your medical care, is your *self-care*:

- Am I getting adequate sleep? Do I make time for rest, vacations? (Sleep and rest deprivation contribute to weight gain.)
- Do I use too much caffeine or alcohol? (For women, limiting alcohol to one drink per day or fewer and

caffeinated beverages to 3 cups a day or fewer are recommended.)

- Do I smoke?
- Is my home organized in such a way that I can find things when I need them? (Clutter and chaos are stressful!)
- Are there aspects of my daily life (my commute, my screen time, my To Do list) that could be altered to reduce my stress?
- Do I live, as much as possible, within my means?
- Do I spend as much time as I can with people I love, doing things that I truly value and enjoy?

The Next Step

How many times have you made the same New Year's resolution ("lose weight," "get in shape," etc.)? One of the reasons these resolutions usually bite the dust before the Valentine's Day flowers have wilted is that they're too big, too vague — too overwhelming.

One technique that professional coaches use to help people set and tackle goals more effectively is the **GROW** model, which I've modified here:

Grab a pen and paper, and write down a **G**oal, based on one of the topics covered in this chapter or, after you've read them, in the coming chapters on eating and exercise. Perhaps you want to get more aerobically fit, get more sleep, eat less saturated fat, or have a more orderly home?

Now, do a **R**eality check. On a scale of 0 to 10, with 10 meaning that you've already achieved this goal and 0 meaning that you feel you've achieved absolutely nothing with regard to this goal, where are you right now? Write that number down.

Time to consider your **O**ptions. Write down the various ways you might try to pursue this goal. What roadblocks do you need to work around? For example, if your goal is to get more aerobically fit, you might start a walking program, or join a pool. If your goal is to get more sleep, a roadblock might be your addiction to late night TV, or caffeinated drinks. Cutting down on saturated fat? Maybe you want to try eating vegetarian dinners more frequently.

Here's where the pedal meets the metal: Write down what you would you need to do to find the **W**ay forward, to move just *one half step* closer to your goal than where you are now. For example, if you scored yourself a 4 on aerobic fitness, how can you get to 4.5? Would getting off the train one stop earlier, or buying a new pair of sneakers, do it? If you need more sleep and you're currently at a 2, would putting your favorite late night show on DVR get you to 2.5? Would looking up a recipe for one meatless dish on the Internet move you from a 5 to a 5.5 in your vegetarian efforts?

You get the idea. And once you've progressed one half step, start the process over again and envision the next half step. You can apply this technique to any kind of goal you have, whether related to healthy eating, stress management—anything!

You'll notice that the women who wrote the stories in this book all accomplished their goals by taking small, specific, manageable steps, one at a time: signing up for an exercise class, eliminating sugary drinks, making the decision to stop talking about diets. You can make similar steps forward. The late tennis champion, Arthur Ashe, once offered some succinct and helpful advice: "Start where you are. Use what you have. Do what you can."

Newly Hip

When I turned sixty, my aching left hip wouldn't let me stand and have a conversation with my neighbors. So, I sat on the stoop. It may have been a bit rude but I chalked it up to aging.

Then my hip wouldn't let me go for long walks, even with a cane. My dog didn't like that but he was aging faster than I was, anyway.

Then, my hip did something I couldn't rationalize away. It refused to let me ride my bike. And it started stabbing me like a knife whenever I took a step. I was an active person. I crawled around on the floor fixing computers for a living. I swam, biked, walked, did yoga and Pilates for fun. My hip wasn't letting me do much more than limp to the bus stop, ride the bus to work, and struggle around on the floor as I did my job.

I went to a sports doctor. I expected exercises, stretches, physical therapy. He did a bunch of muscle testing and then sent me for an MRI. He said my muscles were fine. The problem was my hip. Then he sent me to see an orthopedic surgeon.

The surgeon said, "I won't lie to you. There's no point in giving you a local injection. You need a new hip."

Freak Out City! Like I really wanted somebody to slice me open and install all of that gadgetry. My grandmother did that. She sat around and played cards. I hate playing cards.

I asked the surgeon, "Will I be able to ride my bike?"

He looked at me oddly. "After two weeks, you can ride a stationary bike." Who did he think I was? An old lady? Just because I was in my sixties didn't mean I wanted to ride a stationary bike.

"My real bike," I said.

He looked at me with new respect. "You can ride that after four weeks."

He even promised that he could get the new hip in without cutting any muscles, so I could have a quicker recovery. He'd practiced a new technique for two months on cadavers that uses a short incision on the front of the thigh. I didn't care where the scar was. I wanted to ride my bike!

The surgeon came by to see me a few hours after I woke up from surgery. "Walk as much as possible." I made an appointment to see him in his office in four weeks. He said, "I expect you'll barely be limping by then, but you'll probably still be using a cane."

When I got home from the hospital, I wanted to walk around the block. I couldn't do it. I made it to the corner and back. My neighbors were amazed that I was out of the house. "You were just in the hospital. Stay home. Rest." I didn't want to do that. I didn't want to become a couch potato—not even for a day.

A few days later, I completed my first circuit around the block. My neighbors told me I was a lunatic. And surely my surgeon hadn't meant for me to walk this much this quickly.

A week later, I was walking three blocks to the grocery store. By two weeks, I could walk half a mile to the gym, ride the stationary bike, and walk home. My neighbors stopped telling me

I was pushing myself too hard and started congratulating me on my progress.

I wanted to go farther. Three weeks after the surgery, I asked a friend to meet me at one of our favorite Chinese restaurants. I took the bus, and I allowed myself to use the senior and handicap seats near the front. Those steep stairs on the bus were a struggle, but I'd promised to meet my friend. No way was I going to call her and cancel because of a few stairs.

My friend's hip had begun hurting her. She was going to see an orthopedic surgeon. She was pleased to see me out and about so soon after getting a new hip.

I told her my surgeon's advice: walk as much as possible; ride the stationary bike.

I saw my surgeon after four weeks. He advanced me from the stationary bike to the elliptical and officially gave me permission to start riding my bike. He had me start out on the sidewalk and only take short rides at first.

My friend got a new hip two months after I did. She told me she was the only one on her hospital ward who got a walker and walked the halls just to keep active. She hates stationary bikes. After she went home, she had a physical therapist come to her house to make sure she had the right exercises. And three weeks after her surgery, we met at our favorite Chinese restaurant. She rode the bus and I rode my bike.

Now she has a neighbor whose doctor says she needs a hip replacement. She gave her neighbor my number. Between the two of us, we'll get her out and walking. What's the point of a new hip if you aren't going to use it?

I'm still going to the gym. I've graduated from the elliptical to the cross-trainer and the Helix. Even the gym owner comments on how gracefully I'm walking now. Yes, it does feel like a gadget in there, but that's what it is. A gadget that lets me live my life—my active life.

～ Lois Wickstrom ～

Reunion

"Where in the world did that come from?" When you are sixty-eight years old, looking in the mirror is an adventure. "Where did that wart come from? Was my belly this big yesterday? Is that gray hair coming out of my nose? Are those chin hairs? Is that an eyebrow growing out of the middle of my forehead?"

I've lost weight and gained weight so many times I have five different sizes of clothes in my closet: Skinny, Still Good, Slipping a Little but Still Fits, Oops, Fat Again.

Most of us have lost our waists. We are either straight-up-and-down or we are round. When I was twenty-two years old I had a 22-inch waist. Now I have a 35-inch waist or a 38-inch waist, depending on which roll of fat I measure.

When I received an invitation in the mail for the fiftieth high school reunion for the class of 1961 it made my blood run cold. My old classmates were going to see me fat! When I was in school I was so skinny I got teased. Now they would tease me about being fat.

Oh, yes, and the head of the reunion committee was my arch nemesis in high school, Ginger. Ginger was the cheerleader, class president and most popular girl and she bullied the shy nerds like me.

I'd show them! I would go to the reunion and I would be skinnier than Ginger. I was a woman on a quest; my goal was to look better than Ginger. Of course, I hadn't seen Ginger in fifty years but for some reason I was convinced she still looked like a seventeen-year-old cheerleader.

I would not lose this battle! I took the laundry baskets off my treadmill, dusted it off and began walking on it two hours a day. I stopped eating foods that were bad for me.

I didn't sit and watch TV; I stood to watch TV. I danced, I stacked books on the floor and used them to do step-ups. I didn't walk through the house; I hopped, skipped, jumped and ran through my house. I was in constant motion. Just about the time I thought the pounds were stuck to me with super glue I noticed my clothes were getting loose. My belly looked flatter, my face looked thinner... I was getting a waist!

The date of the reunion was circled on the calendar and I'd written Ginger's name on the date. I had never worked so hard to lose weight so quickly and it was paying off.

Three weeks before the reunion I had reached my goal and had lost thirty pounds. I felt good! I'd show them! I'd show Ginger!

Then I remembered that I'd been terribly unhappy in school. I'd been lonely and unpopular and invisible. After graduation no one in the class had made any effort to contact me and I'd never made an effort to keep in touch with them.

I'd just spent the last two months obsessed with losing weight to look good for a reunion I didn't want to go to so I could impress a woman I'd never liked.

It was so funny I laughed. Ginger hadn't liked me fifty years ago; she wasn't going to like me now. Did I really think losing thirty pounds was going to make me popular with these people who were now strangers? Was I expecting to be the prom queen of the reunion?

I don't have to prove anything anymore. I've had a good life. I'm successful in my career; I'm proud of my family. Why had I let Ginger reach across the decades and shatter my self confidence and turn me back into the shy teenager eating lunch alone in the cafeteria because no one would sit with her?

I threw the reunion invitation into the trash. I erased the circle around the date and I erased Ginger's name. I erased the class of 1961 from my life. I didn't need their approval. I didn't need them to like me. I didn't need to be fifteen years old again.

I let the wrong thing motivate me to lose weight. I should never have lost weight just to look "good enough" to go to the reunion. I should have done it for myself.

Nevertheless, I had made the choice to eat right, eat less, and exercise. I lost thirty pounds, I tightened up my body, and I increased my stamina and my strength.

I'm happy with the way I look now and I'm going to keep my waist. I can't control the wrinkles, I can't stop getting older, but I can control my weight and I can get stronger. I can let go of the past and I can let go of the people who hurt me and made my childhood so unhappy.

I can do all of these things for myself. It's all about me, my health, the way I feel, my happiness.

None of this is about Ginger or the class of 1961.

— April Knight —

Exercising Power

The letter arrived in a pristine white business envelope with my doctor's name printed in the upper left corner. There should have been a warning stamped on it to alert me to its life-changing contents.

Dear Gloria,
Your bone density test suggests osteopenia, which is a lower-than-normal bone mineral density and precursor to osteoporosis. Please make an appointment with my office to discuss treatment options.

Stuck behind the typed letter was another sheet of paper printed with the outline of a woman's anatomy, shaded around the hips and knees to indicate potential "hot spots" of porous bones.

I slumped into my chair, stunned and afraid my next step might snap a bone. I closed my eyes and tried to shut out the memory of my mother's incessant pain from collapsed vertebrae and my grandmother's broken hip. Both suffered the consequences of osteoporosis.

There must have been a mistake. I'd always been healthy. Thin-framed with long, lean limbs. I weighed only 128, a mere eighteen pounds more than my freshman year in college, almost forty years earlier. Who else can say that? I protested to the health gods.

Yet it was time to face the reality I had ignored—I was getting older. I had trusted that exercising three times a week while eating lean meat, fresh fruit and vegetables and avoiding sweets would keep me ageless like Peter Pan. I had only a tiny potbelly where extra weight had settled over my 5'7" frame.

My physician prescribed alendronate to prevent further bone deterioration and suggested weight-bearing exercise along with vitamin D and 1200 mg of calcium per day.

My husband and daughter, the real health nuts in our family, helped me transform my habits. Along with the alendronate and calcium supplements, I drank calcium-enriched orange juice, ate a yogurt daily and choked down broccoli with supper.

Up until this point, I exercised inconsistently after work. More often than not, I was drained of energy by the time I dragged my body through the door and usually just excused myself to assume a couch-potato pose. But now with new resolve, I increased my on-again, off-again exercise sessions to a disciplined thirty minutes every morning before work, five days a week. Two days with weights, Saturday power walks with my husband, and two days with aerobics. I danced with Kathy Smith, ponied with Jane Fonda and marched with Leslie Sansone, all in the name of stronger, healthier bones.

Eight months after launching my mission to prevent further bone loss, my progress came to an abrupt halt. I had to undergo surgery for a twisted colon. Traveling to the emergency room doubled over in severe pain that refused to subside after twenty-four hours, the doctor looked bewildered at the X-rays. He stood at the foot of the bed and matter-of-factly described the diagnosis. I will never forget his concluding pronouncement.

"This happens mainly in older people."

There was that word again... old. My body was aging whether I liked it or not.

Back home, I was restricted for the next eight weeks to walking short distances at a slow pace while I regained strength and stamina. Power protein bars supplemented my meals to accelerate the healing process.

Another two months later, I returned to my doctor for an annual check-up, including the bone density test to determine progress. I worried that the interruption of surgery unraveled any advance I'd made against osteopenia.

The letter arrived a week later in the same pristine white business envelope. I slid my fingers under the flap and braced for the results.

Dear Gloria,

Your osteopenia is stabilized. There is no significant change indicated by the bone density test. Some spots are actually more positive. Keep doing what you're doing. It's working.

I Snoopy-danced in victory around the kitchen table, then grabbed the letter again to finish reviewing other test results.

However, your total cholesterol is borderline and above the preferred upper range limit. Please make an appointment to see me and discuss treatment options.

My aging heart sank. I fell victim again to family history. Doctors diagnosed my mother with high cholesterol when she was in her forties. My sister had recently begun medication for the same condition.

Hoping to avoid medication, I bargained. "What do you think about me first trying to drop my cholesterol through diet and exercise? I'm just getting my routines back on track since surgery." Knowing the discipline with which I tackled osteopenia, my doctor agreed.

I added a sixth day to my workouts and set a goal weight of 120 pounds. My husband, who was the cook in our family, modified our meals. For lunch, frozen meals with cholesterol-producing high saturated fat became turkey sandwiches and carrots along with the usual apple and banana. I sacrificed two squares of Ghirardelli's dark chocolate in exchange for one peanut butter cracker sandwich for a mid-morning snack. Chicken, turkey, and salmon (the only fish I tolerated) showed up for dinner instead of red meat. My husband even prepared spaghetti sauce with ground turkey rather than hamburger, a surprisingly tasty change. I cut about 300 calories out of my daily diet.

An article on the Internet about cholesterol-busting foods prompted further adjustments to my eating habits. Breakfast became a concoction of high-fiber cereal, organic blueberries and seven or eight walnuts, all sprinkled with a teaspoon of ground flax seed. I dipped toasted wheat bread in virgin olive oil with dinner and cut out extra juices that added sugar to my daily intake.

After three months of strictly adhering to the new diet and exercise routine, my weight dropped to 117 pounds, three lighter than goal. I returned to my doctor to determine progress.

A week later, the letter arrived in a pristine white business envelope. I slid my fingers under the flap and braced for the results.

Dear Gloria,

Although still on the high end, your total cholesterol slipped into the allowed normal range, and the ratio of HDL to total cholesterol is acceptable. There is no change in your bone density test, indicating the osteopenia is stable.

So, for now, my attack against the "aging body" syndrome continues. I pound the ground with aerobic workouts, stick to foods that prevent fatty build-up, and take calcium supplements. With any luck, I'll exercise power over family history and slide through my seventies, and beyond, fit enough to conquer anything that comes my way.

— Gloria Ashby —

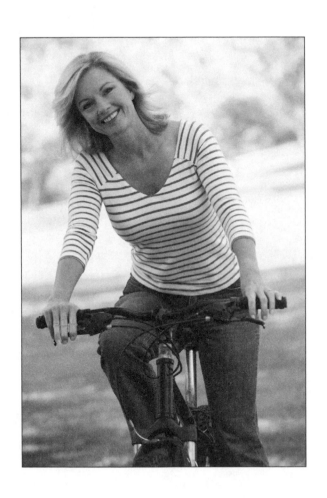

Chapter 3
Moving Forward

Moving Forward

Why Exercise?

When I first read the stories submitted by Chicken Soup for the Soul contributors for this book, I noticed something interesting. Most of the women who lost weight and became fit started out by exercising—often, simply by walking. I have a theory about why this is so. In contrast to dieting, with which so many middle-aged women have a long record of repeated disappointment, exercise has fewer negative associations. Many of us enjoyed playing kickball or jumping rope as girls and, though we may have "sweated to the oldies" with Richard Simmons or "gone for the burn" with Jane Fonda, we are much more likely to have dieted than exercised over the years. This isn't a good thing, of course, but we can use it to our advantage, in that we can now approach exercise and fitness with a fresh point of view.

First, what *is* fitness? It has nothing to do, you'll be relieved to know, with Lycra, spandex, or bulked up muscles. The American College of Sports Medicine (ACSM) defines fitness as follows:

The ability to carry out daily tasks with vigor and alertness, without undue fatigue and with ample energy to enjoy leisure pursuits and to meet unforeseen emergencies.

The ACSM further specifies the different elements of physical fitness, including: fitness of the heart and lungs, muscular strength and endurance, total body fat, flexibility, balance, agility, and reaction time.

In other words, when you're fit, as the women in the stories here describe, you feel more *alive*. You can do more of the things you want and need to do: run around with your grandchildren, plant flowers, hike the Grand Canyon, make love, volunteer in a soup kitchen, change a flat tire, and offer a hand when someone falls. Over fifty, I think most of us find more value (and more motivation) in these things than in "buns of steel."

In addition to feeling better—and, steel buns or not, *looking* better—the health benefits of exercise are incomparable. There is no doctor you can consult, no pill you can take, no surgery you can undergo that can improve your overall physical and mental health more than walking briskly for 30 minutes, five times a week. Does that seem hard to believe? It's not, when you consider the wide range of proven health benefits of regular exercise, summarized here in a 2008 report from the U.S. Department of Health and Human Services:

Strong evidence
- Lower risk of early death
- Lower risk of coronary heart disease
- Lower risk of stroke
- Lower risk of high blood pressure
- Lower risk of adverse blood lipid profile

- Lower risk of type 2 diabetes
- Lower risk of metabolic syndrome
- Lower risk of colon cancer
- Lower risk of breast cancer
- Prevention of weight gain
- Weight loss, particularly when combined with reduced calorie intake
- Improved cardiorespiratory and muscular fitness
- Prevention of falls
- Reduced depression
- Better cognitive function (for older adults)

Moderate to strong evidence
- Better functional health (for older adults)
- Reduced abdominal obesity

Moderate evidence
- Lower risk of hip fracture
- Lower risk of lung cancer
- Lower risk of endometrial cancer
- Weight maintenance after weight loss
- Increased bone density
- Improved sleep quality

So, to re-cap: exercise makes you look and feel better, makes you live longer, makes you less likely to get cancer, a hip fracture, heart disease, depression, diabetes and dementia... and, did I mention, it's fun?

What Kind? How Long? How Strenuous?

If we all still did agricultural work, as many of our ancestors did, we wouldn't have to worry about exercise. We would spend all day walking, bending, reaching, and lifting heavy loads. One study, in which Amish people (who don't use many labor-saving devices) were given pedometers to wear, offered an eye-opening perspective on this. Amish women, just in the course of a day on the farm, walked *five times* the amount currently recommended by the ACSM. What's more, the Amish women didn't decrease the amount they walked as they aged.

Most of us don't work on farms. But we can use various kinds of exercise to achieve all the different types of fitness. In 2011, the ACSM updated its guidelines for adults, summarized here:

Cardiorespiratory Exercise ("Cardio")

Engage in **moderate intensity** exercise 30 minutes per day, on five days per week, for a total of 150 minutes per week. Moderate intensity activities include walking briskly (>3.0 mph), mowing the lawn, dancing, performing yard work, recreational swimming, light rowing, and cycling. Moderate-intensity activity typically causes a light sweat and makes you breathe hard enough so that you are still able to talk, but not sing.

Engage in **vigorous intensity** cardiorespiratory exercise training for 20 minutes per day on three days per week, for a total of 60 minutes per week. Vigorous-intensity activities include race walking, jogging, running, heavy rowing, cycling uphill, swimming laps, and singles tennis. You work up a good sweat and cannot easily carry on a conversation while doing these activities.

You can mix and match these activities, and you don't need to do the recommended time all at once. For example, at the gym you might choose to do 10 minutes each on the treadmill, elliptical, and stationary bike. Or, you can walk for 10 minutes in the morning, 10 minutes after lunch, and 10 minutes after dinner. Or, wear a pedometer and try to walk 3000 steps in 30 minutes, or 1000 steps in 10 minutes three times throughout the day, five days per week. And remember, these are goals to strive for: when you start, you may not be able to walk more than a block or two — that's okay! Little by little, day by day, much sooner than you'd think, you'll reach the recommended targets.

Get creative about sneaking some extra exercise into your day. Park farther than you need to, get off the bus or train a stop early, offer to meet a friend or colleague for a walk instead of coffee. Also, consider using your cardio as a form of meditation. As you walk on the street, track, or treadmill, be aware of your breathing, the swing of your arms, the strike of each footstep. You'll be amazed at how mentally refreshing this is — though it works better if you aren't watching CNN or *Real Housewives* or blasting music through your earphones while you're exercising.

A final note about cardio: the guidelines are for health, not weight loss or maintenance. Participants in the National Weight Control Registry who've maintained at least a 30-pound weight loss for a year or more walk an average of 11,000-12,000 steps a day — that's about five or six miles, four times the ACSM recommendation. If you're serious about losing weight and keeping the weight off, the truth is you'll have to get serious about moving more.

Strength Training

Two to three days a week, perform resistance exercises for each of the major muscle groups. Resistance training can be done with free weights, weight or resistance machines, elastic bands (such as Thera-bands) or with floor exercises such as pushups, sit-ups, and Pilates. Increasing muscle strength boosts metabolism, helps prevent osteoporosis, and reduces back and joint pain. A personal trainer can help you develop a strength-training program (sometimes in just a couple of sessions) or you can use one of the many excellent videos and "on demand" TV exercise programs. "Strong Women Stay Young" (book, video, or class) is a simple and popular 20-minute strength training routine using inexpensive wrist and leg weights.

Flexibility and Balance

Two to three days a week, engage in activities such as yoga, ballet, t'ai chi, or qi qong that improve flexibility and balance. These activities reduce the likelihood of falling—a major health risk as women get older—and are particularly good for reducing stress.

These recommendations may seem time-consuming, but remember, they are targets. Some weeks you may not be able to do everything. Also, some activities can be combined. At the gym, use the cardio equipment before and after lifting weights. Map out a half-hour walk near the yoga studio. With a little planning, you can devise a manageable and enjoyable exercise program that includes most of these activities.

In addition to increasing exercise, studies show it's also important to reduce the time you spend being sedentary. Most people are horrified to learn that the average American child now spends at least seven hours a day in front of TV, computer, and video games. Would you believe that the average baby boomer spends *nine and a half hours daily* in front of a screen? Get into the habit of taking a break from your desk, reading in the evenings instead of watching TV, and limiting your Internet surfing. Even if you're not exercising, almost anything you do will burn more calories than staring at a screen.

Staying Injury-Free

Don't get hurt while getting fit! Injuries are painful and disabling, and they also interrupt your fitness program. Here are a few tips to avoid injury:

- Have the proper equipment: High quality athletic shoes made for your sport (tennis, running, and walking sneakers are all made differently), a bike helmet, and reflective clothing are crucial for injury prevention. Thousands of walkers, joggers, and cyclists are hit by cars every year, many because motorists can't see them.

- Stretch: It used to be thought that stretching before exercise was important. Newer research suggests that it's better to stretch *after* you're warmed up, during or following your exercise routine. Stretching improves flexibility, which, along with improved balance, prevents falls, twisted ankles, and muscle pulls.

- Stay hydrated: Exercise causes you to lose much more body fluid than you think, especially in hot weather. Drink plenty of water and, if it's very hot or you're exercising for an extended period, add some salty and sugary food (like trail mix), a sports drink, or an energy bar.

- Don't ignore pain and fatigue: Your workout should be challenging, not painful or exhausting. If exercise leaves you hurting or wiped out, you may be doing too much too soon (especially after an injury or hiatus) or using improper form (especially when lifting weights). Slow down, ease up, get advice from a trainer or instructor. Dizziness, significant shortness of breath, and chest pain are symptoms for which you should seek immediate medical help.

Making Time for Exercise

The number one reason people give for not exercising is lack of time. And yet, when I ask my patients if they could find the time to take a family member to a daily 30-minute medical appointment, they say "sure!" (In fact, they also admit they'd find the time to take the family dog to a daily 30-minute appointment!)

Some tips for making time to exercise include.

- Mark down your weekly exercise plan—noting specific times—in your calendar. Make an unbreakable appointment with yourself.

- Meet a buddy—human or canine—for your daily walk. Or have a regular meeting time with a buddy or trainer at the gym. You're more likely to show up when someone is expecting you. Several stories in this book, including "My Walking Buddy," "Running Like Sixty," and "The Silver Streakers," attest to this.

- Exercise early in the day. This isn't for everyone but, frankly, it works for most people. I tell my patients that working out in the morning is like having savings taken automatically out of your paycheck, rather than waiting until later to see "what's left over." A morning workout primes your metabolism and makes you more energized and alert all day.

Consider this: There are three phases to each exercise session: before, during, and after. Everyone likes the "after"—you feel good after you exercise. And most people would say that once they're warmed up, they enjoy the "during"—the exercise itself. What nobody likes is the "before"—the thinking about exercise. So don't think about it too much. Have a plan, and "just do it"—there's nothing better for your waistline, heart, lungs, bones, brain, mood, and mind.

Raising the Barre

I knew this would not be a typical ballet class when I looked down the row of ballerinas in pink tights and black leotards and saw several with gray hair. One or two had the posture, taut muscles, and lifted chins of the younger students. Others, like me, bulged in places.

Could a fifty-eight-year-old woman—devastated by mononucleosis for the past year, out-of-shape, and overweight—do ballet? Did I want to?

Yes. After weeks of lying in bed, I decided to take up ballet. I bought an exercise video put out by the New York City Ballet in which a soothing man's voice led me gently through stretches, pliés (slight knee bends), relevés (raising up on the toes), and tendus (pointing the toe out to the side) with lots of additional floor exercises before some final leaps and then relaxing steps. All this movement was done with classical music in the background. Starting out slowly, doing only the first few stretching sections on the tape, I built up to following the dancers through the whole hour.

I soon saw the unique advantages of ballet for the aging body. The slow stretches elongated my limbs and joints and kept me flexible. Most of the steps were traditional positions that emphasized the correct form rather than speed and power.

This helped me focus on controlling my muscles, not just using them. Standing on one foot, while lifting the other, helped with balance. And a surprising bonus was that learning the steps helped my memory.

When I wanted to move beyond the basic steps on the tape, I found a low-impact ballet class for adults in my town. Would they let me in? Yes, if I bought the uniform and paid my money.

Unlike the tape, this class offered the advantage of a long bar, known as a barre. It ran the length of the room, about waist-high. The "disadvantage" was that it faced a wall of mirrors.

We lined up sideways against the barre with one hand on it, all facing the same direction. I shyly stepped to the back of the line. The teacher, Ms. Jones, turned on the traditional ballet music with beats we should follow to be in sync, and led us through the basic foot positions and arm placement, sometimes linking the two into actual dance sequences. However, to my aging ears her voice blended in with the loud music and echoes of moving feet on a solid floor. I found myself mostly following the woman in front of me. Then we turned. Instead of hiding at the back of the line, I was now at the front! I really was lost. I'm sure the woman behind me did not try to follow my steps. Ms. Jones soon moved me to the middle of the line.

This experience made me realize that the live class had a big advantage over the tape. I had to think because I didn't know what was coming. I also had to concentrate on the beats of the music. I had memorized the dancers' movements on the tape and became adept at them. Now, I had to learn, move, and listen all at once because the routine changed every class. It was a welcome challenge.

Fortunately, after a few classes, the positions and steps became a little easier. But Ms. Jones did not cut us any slack. Despite the fact that we were never going to become professional ballerinas she insisted we do the steps correctly, just as she did her younger students. I appreciated her attitude. She did not lower her standards because of our age. Nor did she give us a pass for making the effort to simply show up. Of course, she did not expect the impossible. She did not expect us to do splits or dance on pointe. However, she would physically take my foot and say, "You can do better than that! You have very good feet for ballet. POINT your toes," as she pushed them farther than they had planned to go. Other students, too, found their knees pushed higher than they had meant to lift, or arms guided to the proper angle.

As the semester progressed, I began to know the other students. One lady in her seventies said, "I started taking ballet for my arthritis and neck problems several years ago. It helps so much." Her years of practice showed in her posture and lifted chin. Another woman in her thirties or forties said, "I take classes while my children are in theirs. It really helps with the stress and gives me some time for myself." The most surprising comment came from a strikingly beautiful young woman in her twenties with a perfect body and face. At her age, I was exhausting myself doing two aerobic classes or competing on the tennis court. She said, "I love this class. It's the perfect workout. I leave feeling I've had just the right amount of exercise."

By the end of the year, I felt fitter, more flexible, and healthier from the physical exercise. And I was uplifted by expressing myself in an art form while striving for a goal set at a high "barre."

— Joan Hetzler —

Row Strong, Live Long

I tried once again to zip and button the only pair of jeans I could even attempt to get on. Each time I washed them and they shrank, I would feel discouraged and ashamed. Then they would stretch as I wore them, and I'd be back in my world of denial until the next time I washed the pants and tried to zip and button.

"How did I get this way?" I would cry out at the face in the mirror. I had the answer—years of neglect. At fifty-two years of age, I was at my highest weight ever. My doctor was warning me to lose weight and start taking better care of myself before I began to have more problems. I was already taking medication for high blood pressure and high cholesterol, and my blood sugar was getting too high.

I knew she was right. I did want to live a long, productive, active life. I did want to be able to get on the floor and play with my grandchildren. I did want to be able to do things and go places without always getting out of breath—even if it was only to the grocery store.

Looking into the mirror at my moon face, puffy eyes, and the muffin top spilling over my too-tight jeans, I made a decision. Now was the time. I'd been an athlete during high school and college and knew I was still the same person who enjoyed the thrill of pushing myself to the limit, the feeling of exhaustion after working hard, and the gratification of seeing results. I only had to find something I could do at my age and start doing it.

Walking—I'd tried it the summer before but got discouraged. Weight lifting—I couldn't get excited about working out with weight-lifting machines or free weights as I had in younger years. Spin class—an old basketball knee injury kept me from being able to endure the intense workout. Aerobic class—the knee injury again, too much impact. Water aerobics—wasn't I a little too young? I had an excuse for every activity.

Eventually I ran across an advertisement for an indoor rowing class in a health publication and was intrigued. I'd tried rowing machines in my early twenties, but a class for indoor rowing, conducted like a spin class, sounded fun. As I read the benefits of indoor rowing on their website, I was even more interested. No impact—good for my bad knee. Builds long, lean muscle mass—definitely needed that. Complete upper and lower body workout—not getting any kind of workout at the moment. Relieves stress—now we're talking. Ultimate calorie burning exercise—sounding better and better. Very efficient workout that allows one to accomplish more in less time—sold!

By the next week I was in my first class. With my foot straps tightened, damper setting adjusted, water and towel within reach—I was ready to go. Or was I? Could I keep up with the others? Would I be totally embarrassed if I couldn't? Would I be the largest woman in the class? Could I lean over far enough and pull hard enough? Could I push with enough strength to get any results? Would I pass out?

As the questions ran through my mind I caught sight of my reflection in the mirror in the front of the room. I saw my moon face, puffy eyes, and the muffin top spilling over my too-tight workout pants and remembered my decision. Now was the time. As I looked into the mirror I willed myself to just start—no matter how out of place I felt, how difficult it was going to be, or how long it took me to get the hang of it—just start. If I couldn't row for a long time and keep up, I'd try harder the next day and then the next. I just had to start.

That was fourteen months, two million meters, two half marathons, thirty pounds, and three sizes ago. I've had many encouraging compliments, but the biggest thrill is what I've been able to do. I've had the opportunity to row with the Clemson University rowing club on the lake and will begin training to compete at the Atlanta Erg Sprints. I'm completely off of my blood pressure and cholesterol medicines, have no blood sugar issues, and I feel better than I have in years. I've been so excited about my newfound love of indoor rowing, I take any and every opportunity to tell others. If someone comments on how much weight I've lost or how I look, I tell them about indoor rowing. If someone says they need to start exercising, I tell them about indoor rowing. If someone wants to lose weight like I have... you guessed it, I tell them about indoor rowing.

Am I where I want to be? No, but I'm not where I was either. Getting fit at any age can be done with determination and commitment, but the key is to find something you enjoy doing and start doing it. It's never too late. For me, it's indoor rowing. I plan to, as my coach says, "row strong, and live long." And the moon-face, puffy-eyed, muffin-top lady in the morning rowing class? That lady is no longer there.

— Beth K. Fortune —

My Walking Buddy

"Why don't you take Buddy?" my husband suggested.

I looked at him like he was crazy. He just didn't get it. "Buddy's a dog. I'm talking about a human walking companion."

"Try it. He'd enjoy it," he persisted.

It wasn't the dog's enjoyment I cared about. Truth was, I felt like a slug. I'd been complaining about losing the walking companion I'd had before we got married and moved away. I remembered how happy I'd been to finally find someone to walk with, when I first began an early morning walking routine the previous year. At the age of fifty-six, my metabolism was slow, and I needed a kick-start first thing in the morning to get my blood flowing. It was hard to push myself out the door, but the first month I began walking, I'd lost ten pounds and felt much more energetic. Finding a walking companion had kept me on track.

However, in the three months since our marriage, I was eating more and moving less. I felt heavier, slower, and out of shape. I wanted someone to talk with while I walked, knowing conversation made the exercise go faster. Plus, I needed a person to keep me accountable. I had hoped my husband would be my new walking partner, but his work schedule prohibited it. There was no one in our new neighborhood who could walk with me either.

Buddy was my husband's dog, a big, black, flat-coated retriever. We had taken him for walks a few times together and let him run loose through the woods, but not for a walk around the neighborhood.

A dog walking partner wasn't what I had in mind. I won't call myself a "cat person," because I've always had both cats and dogs, but I must admit I thought cats were easier to manage. They were independent (which dog-lovers dislike), they took care of their personal needs by themselves, and all I had to do was feed them or pet them. I'd lived in houses with large, fenced-in back yards, where the dogs we'd had could "walk" themselves. The few times I'd attempted to take them for walks proved unpleasant for both of us. They either balked at the leash and I had to drag them, or they continually went off in the wrong direction. No, I didn't need a dog. I needed a person. Someone with whom I could talk. Someone who would encourage me.

I tried taking walks by myself, but was very inconsistent, as I often got distracted by things around the house before I set out and then didn't have time for a walk. One thing that was consistent however, was Buddy's reaction. Each time I went for a walk, I could hear him barking behind me as he watched me leave.

Finally I decided to give it a try. I walked over to the place where we hung the dog leash and picked it up. When I started towards Buddy with it, he got really excited and started prancing around, eager to go.

"Okay, okay. We'll see how this works," I told him.

I opened the front door and Buddy shot out, running down the driveway and almost jerking the leash out of my hand. He paused to briefly sniff the mailbox, before I pulled him away and we were off.

And so we pressed on, Buddy trotting obediently beside me most of the time. There were a few times, however, that he stopped to check out some inviting aroma, and I continued on unaware until I ran out the length of the leash and almost pulled my arm out of the socket. So much for exercise. Despite the stops, however, it still felt better to get out of the house and move, rather than do no exercise at all.

When I told my husband that evening about the arm-jerking experience, he explained to me that Buddy, who was trained to walk on a leash, could be encouraged to continue by saying, "Let's go," or just tugging on the leash a little when he tried to stop.

Okay, maybe it was worth another try. The next time went better than the first, and Buddy did a better job of keeping pace with me. In fact, with his long legs, I could jog while he barely trotted. Of course, there were still a couple of times that Buddy found some scent simply irresistible, and I was forced to wait until he was ready to move on again. Overall, though, the experience was not so bad.

I decided that I would take him occasionally, and other times go it alone. However, anytime I put on my tennis shoes,

Buddy started getting excited and expected to go for a walk. Guilt attacked my conscience when I went without him and let him down. Buddy started coming into the bedroom as soon as I got up, eagerly imploring me with his eyes, "Are we going for a walk this morning?" Of course, I had to take him; he was so eager to go.

And so it began—Buddy "dogging" my steps every morning until I took him for a walk. Pretty soon we had a routine. Together we explored the neighborhood, discovering interesting trails. Buddy met other dogs and their people, and I learned to enjoy the scenery, observing birds and flowers along the path, especially when Buddy stopped to check out a fascinating new scent.

I discovered other things to enjoy, too, like singing (when we were alone in the woods and I wouldn't frighten anyone). I also found that I could spend the time meditating and praying. And occasionally, I talked to Buddy, who never argued or disagreed.

Buddy became my walking companion, keeping me consistent and re-establishing my exercise routine. Both of us benefited, as neither of us was getting any younger. Buddy, age fourteen, needed the exercise to keep his joints from stiffening up, and I needed the exercise for my mental and physical health. And so I found a new walking buddy to help me stay in shape. And he's not a bad listener, either.

~ Marilyn Turk ~

Keep It Steady

The mirror didn't lie. I needed to lose weight. Tone up. Get stronger. Feel better. Waist? What waist? It didn't exist. My chin had doubled and my upper arms jiggled. Even my legs, my best feature, looked flabby. I'd just passed my fifty-second birthday and my daughter's wedding was only months away.

"Have you picked out your dress for the wedding, Mom?" That was my daughter's first question when she had called the previous evening.

I hesitated. I'd already gone to a bridal shop to look at mother-of-the-bride dresses, but I hated to admit to Katy that I was appalled at the size of the dresses that fit me. I hadn't tried on a dress in years and now I knew why.

"Not yet," I hedged. "I'll know when I find the just the right dress."

JOIN JAZZERCISE NOW! The ad in the morning paper was printed in bright red and went on to describe a sixty-minute program that promised a cardiac workout complete with strength training and toning. I wasn't excited about dancing around in my old sweats with a bunch of twenty-year-old girls in their tight little leotards. Wouldn't it be easier to exercise at home in front of the television? That's what I used to do when I wanted to exercise. Jane Fonda and I were practically best friends.

But now my husband worked a rotating shift at the lock and dam. Towboats push barges through the locks at any time of day or night. Joe's schedule kept changing. While I didn't work the shifts with him, his hours began to have an impact on me. Insomnia plagued me and my lack of sleep began to show as I went about my days in a general haze of sluggishness. I couldn't remember the last time I'd actually exercised.

I knew I needed to make changes in my life. Not only was my body out of sync, but my spiritual life, my inner sense of wellbeing, was suffering too. I was too hazy to read my morning devotionals as well.

I glanced at the paper again. The morning Jazzercise class began in half an hour. Before I could change my mind, I found an old T-shirt and shorts, grabbed a pair of tennis shoes and headed out the door.

"Okay, ladies! Are you ready to work harder?" Kristal, the Jazzercise instructor, jogged to the middle of the stage, snapping her fingers in time to the music.

I felt like I had been working hard for hours, but I knew it had only been ten minutes. Sweat already beaded my forehead and I gulped water from my bottle. Suddenly, I wasn't so confident about my latest decision to get fit. I couldn't understand the words from the contemporary songs that blasted from the speakers and the dance steps were much faster than I had anticipated.

"Whew!" I commented to the gal next to me as we took a break before the strength training. "I don't know if I can make it!"

She was about my age and I was relieved to note that most of the ladies in the morning group were middle-aged. No teeny-tiny twenty-year-olds in this group, although many of them were in super shape. Toned arms, flat tummies. And the smiles on their faces! Everyone seemed to be in a great mood.

"Of course you can," she said. "It gets easier. You've got to keep coming, that's all. Keep it steady."

After the weight training, we stretched to a slow song and my muscles almost shouted out loud in pleasure.

Class ended as we all clapped for our instructor. "Good class. You guys are great!" Kristal applauded us, too. "See you tomorrow!"

"Are you coming back?" the gal who had stood next to me asked as I wiped sweat from my face with a towel.

Another lady stopped me at the door. "Did you enjoy the class?"

I had never met these ladies, but they were so welcoming, so kind.

"Sign me up," I said to Kristal. "I'll be here tomorrow."

The next class was still difficult and my muscles were pretty sore from the day before. My heart still pounded and I felt pretty awkward as I watched the other participants out of the corner of my eye.

Geez, I thought. Some of these gals could be professional dancers.

Another song, another set of dance steps. Despite my breathlessness, despite my inability to keep up, a reluctant grin crossed my face. This was a song I actually knew and I was beginning to find a pattern in the choreography.

"Chasse, step, step," Kristal chanted to the music. "Back again, chasse, step, step."

A childhood memory flitted through my mind as I remembered from my dance class days that a chasse meant one foot chased the other. I glided my left foot after my right and swung my arms in rhythm. I step, stepped. I was dancing! I'd truly forgotten how much I loved to dance. For a moment, I felt almost overwhelmed by the sheer joy of moving my feet to the beat of a song. Bliss. Pure bliss.

"Keep it steady," my new friend advised me again that day. "Don't stop coming."

Maybe it was the endorphins that kicked in after class. Or the songs I continued to hum in my car on the way home. Perhaps it was the encouragement from Kristal and the other ladies. But I hadn't felt this good, both in mind and body, since my husband started his rotating shift work.

I was getting my life back in order. By staying true to my Jazzercise schedule, I was able to keep myself on track. I slept better, I was more careful about my diet, and my morning devotional time became richer.

"Have you found a dress yet, Mom?" Katy sounded a bit worried. "You're running out of time. What if you have to get it altered?"

I was in my bedroom when she called and I smiled into the mirror. I'd lost a couple of inches off my waist, one of those chins had disappeared, my legs looked great and my arms were toned. Keeping it steady had really worked.

I'd found a dress two days earlier. It was a navy blue sheath with a bolero jacket and it was two whole sizes down from the last time I'd tried on dresses.

"I picked up a dress the other day," I said happily. "It's perfect. Absolutely perfect. The only alteration it needs is the hem. I think it's time for your mom to show off her legs!"

— Monica Morris —

Running Like
Sixty

Not long before my sixtieth birthday, I took stock. I'd been working for the Ministry of Education in the idyllic Republic of Seychelles for two years. On sunny weekends I'd flop on a lounge chair at the Coral Strand Hotel on Beau Vallon beach and read Jane Austen. On rainy weekends I'd slump on the aquamarine sofa in my miniscule condo in the hilltop community of Saint Louis, and read Charles Dickens.

Unfortunately, reading doesn't burn up many calories. I'd convinced myself that a twenty-minute stroll down the hill to the beach, and a slightly more arduous climb back, constituted a solid exercise regime. Sadly, those ambles, even coupled with occasional splashes in the warm Indian Ocean, hadn't countered my frequent splurges in takeaway fish curries, savory samosas, and ginger bananas.

Now my hibiscus-patterned one-piece Catalina bathing suit threatened to burst at the seams. When I hopped on the scales at the Youth Health Centre, I didn't remain there long enough to convert from kilometers to pounds. Horrified, I realized I'd segued from comfortably padded to uncomfortably overstuffed.

If I truly sought to be trim and fit, I'd heard of one

possible resource. For months I had read announcements in the *Seychelles Nation* about the activities of the Hash House Harriers. The Harriers, which advertised itself as a drinking club with a running problem, originated with Brits in 1938 in Kuala Lumpur, Malaysia, to promote physical fitness and conviviality. I'd heard that the Harriers boasted hundreds of chapters in dozens of countries.

My British friend, Heather, twenty years my junior, who worked at the National Archives, had told me that the Hash was the one place in Seychelles where locals, ex-pats, social butterflies, the occasional tourist, and even bona fide athletes, could mingle for some inexpensive fun on this outrageously pricey island. But running? Me?

Heather's boyfriend, Nigel, who managed the BBC Relay Station, ran regularly with the group. She went along to help set up refreshments for the "On In," the party at the end of the trail. Though she hadn't participated yet, she intended to join the pack soon, and encouraged me to accompany her.

She provided more details. The trails, eight to ten kilometers long, were laid out in advance by those familiar with the Seychelles granitic terrain. No two were ever alike. They started at different points on Mahé Island, and often included false detours through the jungle, shortcuts through tea plantations, dead ends, and splits.

"All those stops and starts help keep the pack together," Heather said. "Nigel says that even the fast front-runners have to slow down to find the real trail."

I pictured myself wilting through the bush in the tropical

heat and humidity, forced to forage for fallen star fruit for subsistence. That lounge chair at the Coral Strand seemed much more inviting. I could be there on Saturdays instead, rereading *Sense and Sensibility*.

"I'd probably lag so far behind everybody else that I'd be lost forever."

"That won't happen," Heather said. "We can't use that as an excuse not to try. They always have a designated sweeper, a person who remains with the last group of runners and walkers so even the slowest gets safely back."

I relented. Heather and I became Harriettes. At first some more experienced Harriers teased us about belonging to "The Knitting Circle," a mildly derogatory term for those who spent more time walking and talking than actually running. For the first several weeks Heather and I usually limped in near the back of the pack, lurching thirstily towards the tubs of iced soda and SeyBrew, the local beer.

Then Heather hit upon a strategy to toughen us up so we could actually run part of the trail, or at least the downhill parts.

"There's a new exercise group meeting at the football stadium. They have some bending and stretching exercises first, and then everybody runs around the track. We can start building up some stamina."

"Heather, I'm fifty-nine years old," I cried. "I'm never going to be able to run around the stadium."

"Well, I'm not nineteen and I don't want to do it by myself. Please?"

I just couldn't turn her down. Heather and Nigel had been

generous in inviting me to a Christmas feast of prawn curry cooked in coconut milk at their home at the top of La Misere pass, with its flame-tree shaded patio view of the sparkling turquoise sea. How could I say "no" after that?

Reluctantly, I agreed. Twice a week Heather stopped by the Ministry of Education to meet me, and together we ambled to the stadium. We both relished the stretching exercises, and on one memorable afternoon, I ended up the highest scorer for flexibility. I could still bend over, knees straight, and square my palms flat on the floor in front of my toes.

At first Heather and I cantered together about halfway around the track. Soon Heather sailed ahead, with me falling behind where I could admire the bounce of her blond ponytail. If she lapped me, she would encourage me with the Hash refrain of "on on." I'd smile grimly, wipe the moisture from my face, and keep putting one foot in front of the other.

Finally, one Saturday afternoon, the two of us broke away from "The Knitting Circle" in a tandem trot, to whistles of admiration from the day's sweeper, a rather odiferous gentleman known as Sweaty Teddy. We shot each other conspiratorial smiles, and smugly strode to the next incline, where we slowed once more to a walk.

An hour later we hit what appeared to be the final stretch before our destination at Bel Ombre. We sped up, and scampered into the On In, welcomed by our fellow Harriers, who invited us to join them for a traditional "Down Down," where Harriers were expected to chugalug.

Unlike more serious Hash clubs though, this was a gracious

group who didn't force British or aging American ladies to swill their refreshments. Heather and I were allowed to simply raise our bottles to cries of "cheers," and sip as we mopped our foreheads.

In the spring, Nigel and Heather returned to their home in Southampton. But I remained with the Hash until my departure later that year. By summer I learned that the group planned to stage its first Moonlight Hash on the evening of my sixtieth birthday.

I wish I could brag that I gamboled effortlessly through the Seychelles brush that night, but the truth is I merely plodded and stumbled, waving my flashlight to seek a secure footing. But for the last kilometer, over flatter trail as we neared the On In, to the huzzahs of my companions, I ran like the dickens, ran like greased lightning, ran like the wind.

Yes, indeed. Thanks to Heather and a little perseverance, I ran like sixty!

— Terri Elders —

Water Walking

Losing weight and staying in shape was never an issue in my twenties or even in my thirties. Something changed, however, when I reached my forties. I started to gain weight ever so gradually. Apparently my metabolism had slowed down without me even realizing it. By the time I turned fifty, I weighed forty pounds more than I had at my wedding!

Going to the gym three times a week and walking on the treadmill was helping me maintain my weight, but I wasn't losing any. My wake-up call occurred when I saw a picture of myself and focused on how I had changed. I knew I needed to make a lifestyle change, take control of my weight and overall health, and do it right away.

I'm not exactly sure what contributed to the weight gain, but I probably should not have watched as many cooking shows as I did. The first thing I did was rein in my carbohydrate and sugar intake. Just making a few changes there paid great rewards. I started eating oatmeal for breakfast, snacked on nuts, and incorporated more fruits and vegetables into my diet. Ten pounds vanished pretty quickly, which made me think I was making progress.

I also decided to get a puppy. Taking my little Westie around the neighborhood several times a day definitely keeps me moving. Walking the dog helped, but I knew I needed to do more.

The answer to my exercise dilemma came at the end of May, when our local pool opened. That's when I really stepped up my exercise program. I am proud to now call myself a water walker.

After the pool closes for the day for swimming, it reopens for all the adults who want to water walk. We walk through the pool, which is shaped like a winding lazy river, and is surrounded by flowers and other pools. Upbeat music plays as we march forward with the current or, for the really ambitious, walk against the current.

As you gingerly step into the pool for the first time, you can't help but feel invigorated by the cool water. Walking in the water makes you feel refreshed and reenergized. It is great exercise for everyone since it is low impact. All of your stress from the day just melts away. People of all ages are able to participate and can walk at their own pace. Some jog through the water, some walk really fast, and some just saunter through for the fun of it.

Did I mention that everyone is smiling and laughing? There is a real sense of camaraderie and many new friendships are formed. I have encountered people from all walks of life and enjoy listening to everyone's stories. We always encourage each other to come back the next night and tell each other that we have missed them if they have been away.

I must admit that I am totally addicted to water walking. I walk for the whole session of almost two hours and then take a victory lap by floating in an inner tube. My mood is not nearly as cheerful if I am not able to walk due to schedule conflicts or bad weather. I don't even want to think about the end of the water-walking season. Labor Day weekend signifies the end of summer at the pool and everything closes down. We wish we could ask the park department to build a big bubble around our pool so that we could continue all year. But all good things must come to an end, so we will patiently wait until next May when we can begin again.

Thanks to all of the exercise I am getting, I am pleased to say that I have lost over twenty pounds. How did I lose weight? Diet and water... water walking, that is.

— Kelley Knepper —

Fabulous Fifties

The sound of bagpipes carried me along as I weaved and bobbed my way through the crowds lining Fifth Avenue. St. Patrick's Day can be blustery cold in Manhattan but that year the Irish and nearly Irish of New York were blessed with sunshine and crystalline blue skies. It was a glorious day as I raced to meet friends for drinks. Suddenly I was stopped by an attractive, well-dressed woman.

"Excuse me. Would you be interested in going to an open casting call for L'Occitane?"

Oh sure, like I'm gullible enough to fall for that line. What's she selling?

"A casting call? For what?" I asked.

"L'Occitane," she said proudly, as if I should know the name.

"Sorry, never heard of it. I'm sort of in a hurry."

"L'Occitane," she repeated. "We're having an open casting call today and you have a great look. Do you have an agent?"

A great look? Who, me?

"Never heard of it but you're so sweet to ask," I said. "I really have to go. I'm only in New York for a few days and fly home tomorrow. But please tell me the name of the company one more time so that I can tell my daughters when I get home. They'll be so impressed."

As I continued my race to meet my friends, I wondered if she could possibly have been serious. Had I really just been "discovered," like in the movies? Wait until everyone back home in Colorado heard. Had I really come that far in ten short weeks?

It was early January when I had hit bottom, thoroughly disgusted by how much weight I had gained over the past decade. The weight had crept on slowly, steadily, a pound or two at a time, until nothing in my closet fit. Dressing to go out that Saturday night had turned into a demoralizing series of wardrobe changes, flinging clothes in all directions, trying to find an outfit to hide the dumpy, frumpy fifty-six-year-old woman I had become.

How had this happened? I was of the generation that had pledged to stay forever young. I had spent a good deal of the 1970s braless in halter tops. Now I was wondering where I might buy a girdle. The woman in my mirror was not even close to the woman in my head. One of those images needed to change and I much preferred the one in my head. That night, as I pulled on baggy pants with an elastic waist, topping it off with a shapeless sweater to hide the back fat, I resolved to make some changes. Big changes. Finally. No excuses.

The first step was Weight Watchers. I had used Weight Watchers years ago to lose my post-baby fat. Unfortunately, menopause and the stress of raising teenagers had taken its toll and I had slip-slided my way back to my old, self-destructive eating habits. I found a friend who also wanted to lose weight and we became weight-loss buddies, cheering each other's successes at our weekly weigh-ins.

I wanted to lose at least twenty-five pounds but that

seemed overwhelming. Instead, I focused on just one pound at a time. As long as I lost even half a pound each week, I felt like a success. Nothing succeeds like success. As I lost one or two pounds each week, it became easier to make good choices. I learned that it didn't matter how much I ate but what I ate. Radishes—crisp, spicy and filling—became my favorite snack food. I couldn't live without bread but if I chose whole grain bread with sunflower seeds rather than the white bread I was raised on, I used fewer points and felt full longer. I could choose when and how to splurge, so no food became permanently off limits. I could skip the candy bar on Tuesday, choosing instead to save my bonus points for popcorn and Pepsi at the movies on Saturday. After a week of healthy eating, I felt entitled to lick butter and salt off my fingers in a darkened theater on a Saturday afternoon. After a few weeks of healthy eating, I noticed that I felt better when making good choices and that sugary snacks were not worth the sugar crash that always followed.

The other piece of the puzzle was exercise. Over the years, I had tried them all. Jazzercise hurt my knees. Pilates hurt my shoulder. Zumba left me wishing I could trade some of my German/Irish heritage for even a drop of Latin blood. Cycling made me sweat. I hate to sweat.

I decided to try aqua fitness. You don't sweat when you're in the pool. The buoyancy of the water allows you to jump without any injury to your joints. My local rec center offered aqua fitness classes two mornings a week. I could tolerate anything two mornings a week.

My first encounter with the aqua fitness class won me over. At fifty-six, I was the youngest in the class. Not one Lycra-clad firm body to be seen. The class consisted of women in their sixties, seventies, and eighties. Some had arthritis. Others were recovering from joint replacements. I felt young in their company and couldn't imagine how the class could be very challenging. I was in for a surprise.

Our instructor really knew her stuff, pushing us through exercises that worked every muscle group, every body part. We worked at our own pace, some faster than others. But when I checked my pulse and found it to be 160, I knew I was burning calories. When I returned home an hour later and was too tired to get out of the car, I knew that I had found my ideal workout. I could hop, skip and jump without hurting my knees. I could push myself to my peak endurance without breaking a sweat. And I was surrounded by women twenty years my senior, showing me that age is no excuse to sit on the couch and watch the world go by. I saw my future and it looked to be darn fun.

Between the changes to my diet and regular exercise, the pounds started coming off and I lost thirty-five pounds. I rediscovered my cheekbones and wrists. Friends, and even their husbands, started to comment on the change in me. I decided to take a chance and see if the woman from L'Occitane was right about my "look." I signed with an agent in Denver for the occasional modeling job calling for a white-haired woman.

That's how I came to be standing here, backstage at a fashion show at a local department store. They needed an assortment of models and I was selected as their mature model.

Had I ever done anything like this before? Gosh no. I had to do an Internet search to find clips of runway walks and turns. I practiced walking and turning in heels all week. Was I scared beyond words? You betcha. But there's a first time for everything. And you never know what you can do until you try.

— Carol Britt Bryant —

The Silver Streakers

The year I turned fifty-nine was a terrifying one for me. My mother died of breast cancer at fifty-nine, and as irrational as it is, I never believed I would live past fifty-nine. The entire year I couldn't focus, was depressed, and was overweight. I had lost some weight but hit a plateau. I kept saying, "I can do this on my own," but I just kept cycling through various unsuccessful weight loss attempts. I hated my body.

During that year, I began a sporadic walking routine. In May, I walked in the Race for the Cure in memory of my mother and in September I ran in the Crohn's & Colitis Foundation race in honor of my son-in-law. That was where I met Marjie.

She was a tall blonde in red, white and blue running shorts slightly ahead of me the entire race. I just couldn't catch her. After the race, I asked her to run with me. Marjie was a long-distance runner, nine years younger than me and quite a bit faster. She had been running for many years. In spite of all that, we became running partners. We started meeting twice a week in the park at 7 a.m. Marjie taught me a lot about running. She taught me that the first mile is always hell until your muscles warm up. She taught me to dress for ten degrees warmer than the actual temperature. She taught me that you run even if you don't feel like it because afterwards you will be glad you did.

But more than teaching me tips and tricks, she became my reason for getting out of bed in the morning. Marjie was waiting for me at the bottom of the hill twice a week at 7. I knew she was there so I had to get myself up and going because Marjie wasn't going to be the one to call and say it's too hot or too cold to run. Rain or shine, ice or snow, hot or cold, Marjie wouldn't give up and she wouldn't let me give up.

One December morning I woke up and checked the outside thermometer—it was eighteen degrees! I was sure that Marjie would call and say it was too cold to run. But the call never came. Not wanting to be the wimp, I dutifully donned my tights, woolen pants, thermal underwear, woolen socks, warm sweater, heavy jacket, hat and gloves, and jogged down the hill. Sure enough, there was Marjie wearing a light windbreaker and leggings. The snow on the ground meant we couldn't run our usual dirt and gravel route in the park. Instead, we slowly made our way up the hill where a path had been cleared for cars. We laughed and joked the entire time, marveled at the beauty of the snow-covered trees, admired the breathtaking, top-of-the-hill view of the city garbed in white and giggled at our insane decision to run in eighteen degrees. (And yes, I was overdressed.)

On our runs we shared experiences, hopes, dreams. We talked about books, current events, our jobs, and our husbands. Those forty-five minutes together were quality time. There were no phone calls, interruptions, or distractions. All through that cold, dark winter, Marjie dragged me out for runs.

Then, in April, I turned sixty. I felt like the death sentence had been lifted, like I could start life all over. Outside it was spring; inside my heart spring also came. I promised myself I would do everything I ever dreamed of but hadn't yet. I hired a personal trainer; I entered more races.

Marjie and I continued running through several seasons. One March, at the opening race of the year, a woman flew past me to place first in my age group. I was impressed and asked her to run with us. Thus Pearl joined our running group.

Pearl, white-haired and petite, is three years older than I, and a long-distance runner. Between Marjie and Pearl, they have sixteen marathons under their sneakers! Pearl is always searching out ways to become a better runner. She e-mails us articles on how to breathe from the belly or tells me about great running socks that will solve my foot problem. Pearl suggests different routes or new routines to shake things up a bit.

Pearl is also a breast cancer survivor. I learned from Pearl that your self-talk can make you or break you, that you run with focus and determination, and that while your physical problems may limit you, they don't define you. Whatever happens, she finds the good in it. She has an indomitable spirit.

On our runs we often talk about the joys and sorrows of raising children and grandchildren. Pearl is a sympathetic listener and a woman with the wisdom of experience. When the husband of my dear friend passed away, my running friends were a sounding board and a comfort as we talked, ran, and shared tears and laughter. Sometimes we playfully call ourselves The Silver Streakers!

Some years before I met Pearl, I ran a half marathon in

Philadelphia. It was a horrible experience. I declared I would never do another. Over the course of a couple of years, Pearl and Marjie convinced me to try again. They said they would see to it that I not only got through it but enjoyed it. We picked a training program and for the next five months we trained—hard! In May of 2009, we three Silver Streakers lined up at the starting line (well, okay, we started at the back of the pack) for the Pittsburgh Half Marathon. Crossing the finish line full of exuberance and energy, I was grateful to Marjie and Pearl for enabling me to have an awesome experience.

Several years ago, I decided to enter a triathlon. I was a fearful swimmer and a timid biker. Though by then my running was stronger, I had to complete the swimming and the biking prior to the run. I feared I would pass out on the race-course! I confided in Marjie and Pearl, and their immediate response was: "We'll meet you on the trail and run you in." I was surprised and moved by their unexpected kindness.

The day of the triathlon arrived, bright and early. Marjie and Pearl were there by the pool, cheering me on. Marjie and Pearl were there by the bike course, yelling and applauding. And Marjie and Pearl were there as I jumped off the bike, and with rubber legs, started out on the trail for the race. They ran with me to the finish line. I came in last in the triathlon, but they came in first in my heart.

Marjie and Pearl are my role models. They have challenged, supported, motivated, changed, and inspired me.

I'm very rarely depressed now. I'm trim and fit. I am happy

with my body. But I couldn't do it alone. I am only able to succeed through the kindness and caring of my Silver Streaker
friends.

~ Simone Sheindel Shapiro ~

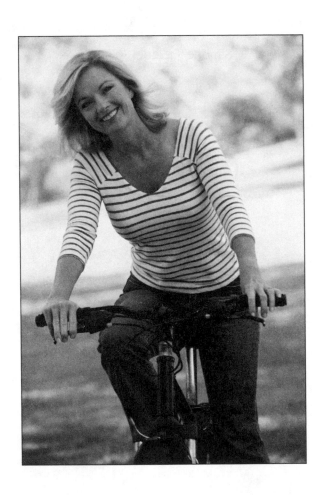

Chapter 4
Food for Thought

Food for Thought

What Should I Eat? And How Much?

A patient of mine, a middle-aged woman who struggles with her weight, once told me that she drove to the supermarket but found herself in tears in the parking lot, unable to get out of her car. "Why?" I asked. "Because I just don't know what I'm supposed to eat!" she answered. How did food, such a basic and pleasurable thing, get so anxiety-provoking?

However it happened, we can certainly say *when* it happened: sometime between the childhoods and adulthoods of the women reading this book, eating got very complicated. As Americans and others in the developed world became heavier, dieting became a multi-billion dollar industry — and a cacophony of conflicting advice, much of it shouting from food labels, resulted. 99% Polyunsaturated! Low Carb! Organic! Sugarless! More Fiber! High in Calcium! And, my favorite: "Fat Free Half-and-Half." (When you figure that one out, please let me know.)

No wonder my patient broke down in front of the supermarket.

Things used to be simpler. People ate less, weighed less, and obsessed about food less. Whether or not you grew up in a rural area, eating home-canned fruits and vegetables, I'm sure you'll relate, as I did, to the story "The Tiny Waist of the Fifties," that you'll read later in this chapter. When we were kids, people ate smaller portions, less processed food, less refined sugar, less restaurant and takeout food, and more meals with their families. Plus, they dieted less, walked more, took more vacation time, and spent far fewer hours staring at screens. And—no surprise—they were, on average, much thinner than adults today. Since the late 1970's, the prevalence of obesity among adults in the United States has doubled. Two out of three Americans are now overweight, and one out of three is obese. If this trend isn't slowed or reversed, it's estimated that *half* of all Americans will be obese by 2030—with disastrous consequences for our national health and economy.

Take a little trip down memory lane to get a more personal sense of how changes in lifestyles have contributed to our society's weight problem. What and how did you eat when you were a kid? Were you physically active? What did the adults around you look like? In my 1960's childhood we had dinner as a family almost every night; I drank Coca-Cola (in a 6-ounce bottle) only at birthday parties and other special occasions; my parents allowed me to watch TV for one hour on Sunday evening (*The Wonderful World of Disney!*); I walked to school, home for lunch, back to school, and home again (about a mile and a half, total, every day)—and very few of my teachers, or the ladies who worked in the beauty parlor, the bank, and the drugstore, or my mom's friends or my friends' moms... were obese!

But while we can take a few pointers from our mothers'

more svelte lifestyle, nostalgia isn't the total solution to our current weight and fitness challenges. There are certain realities of modern life with which we have to contend: two-career families, long commutes, an endless supply of labor-saving devices, computers, and other gadgets that encourage us to be sedentary, and fattening food tempting us at every turn. It's just not practical, and probably not even desirable to most of us, to turn back the clock to the June Cleaver era. Plus, we can benefit from the enormous amount of information that researchers have learned about nutrition and health in the past few decades.

Before I get to specific recommendations about how and what to eat in order to lose weight and stay healthy, it's important to say something you've likely already figured out from long experience: *Diets don't work.* You've been told this time and again — often in the first sentence of a new diet book! And the more restrictive a diet is, the more types of foods it prohibits, the more likely it is to fail.

There's a good reason for the dismal track record of virtually all diets — and, no, it's not that we lack willpower. Psychologists at the University of Rochester have observed that one of the most powerful human drives is our desire to be independent. That makes sense, from a biological perspective. Though we live in families and communities, we also need, as individuals, to fend for ourselves to survive. The rebellious behaviors of two-year-olds, teenagers, and even elderly people whose independence is threatened, reflect the natural resistance we humans have to being told what to do. A diet plan that someone else has prescribed — whether it's the author of the latest weight loss book, your doctor, or a well-meaning relative, tends to bring out the rebel in you. As you "break" your diet, gorging on "forbidden" foods, there's a part of you that's thumbing your nose and saying "So *there*!" It's much more effective to gather information about exercise and healthy eating, such as you'll find here, and figure out what suits your tastes and lifestyle best. If you're the boss, that inner rebel will have much less reason to rebel.

There are some people who lose weight and even keep that weight off with commercial or medically supervised diet programs, but I've noticed that my patients who have stuck with such plans have found ways to personalize them so that they don't feel like they're "following orders." The National Weight Control Registry, the research database that tracks people who've maintained at least a 30-pound weight loss for one year or longer, shows that people are just as likely to be as successful devising their own weight loss plans as following a formal program. "The Tiny Waist of the Fifties," "The Closet Witch," "The Power of Four," and "An Apple a Day" are all stories that show how effective a DIY food plan can be for weight loss.

Additionally, an important study published in the *New England Journal of Medicine* in 2009 showed that low fat diets and low carbohydrate diets were equally effective in helping people lose weight, as long as calorie intake was reduced.

Bottom line: the only thing that makes you lose weight is burning off more calories than you take in, with a 3500 calorie deficit required to lose one pound. True, age, heredity, hormones, and other issues can affect your metabolism (the rate at which you burn calories with routine activity) but, by far, the two most important factors in weight loss are how many calories you consume, and how many you burn off.

Now to some specifics: If you are moderately active (exercising 30 minutes per day), you need to eat about 15 calories per pound to maintain your weight. So, multiply your current weight by 15. Then subtract 250 calories a day for a half pound weight loss per week (500 calories for 1 pound per week). As you lose weight, the number of calories you need to maintain your weight goes down, so you have to keep adjusting your intake.

For example, if you are now maintaining a weight of 200 pounds, then eating roughly 3000 calories a day keeps you there. Along with daily exercise, eliminating just 250 calories a day—that's a slice of pizza, a brownie, a 20-ounce soda, or a large whole milk latte—will result in a 25-pound weight loss over a year!

Does this mean that if you eat nothing but jelly beans and French fries you'll lose weight, as long as you don't eat too many of them? Well… yes. But you'll feel awful and invite all sorts of health problems—not a great strategy for long-term success. The optimal goals, especially important for women over fifty, are to reduce calories and eat foods that promote health and prevent disease. Fortunately, these two goals are very compatible and, in many ways, easier to achieve than ever, because of the wide variety of nutritious foods now available.

So forget diets—you've given them a good try, over many

years, and they haven't yielded lasting results, right? It's time for something new. Here are five simple and flexible guidelines that sift through all the confusing information out there and give you just what you need to know to make your own plan to lose weight and get healthier—for good.

1. Eat Less

Obvious? Perhaps, but, along with "move more," this is the most helpful and honest weight loss advice anyone can give you. Many of my overweight patients actually eat mostly healthy food, they just eat too much of it. That's easy to do, since portions are so much larger than they were even a generation ago. Sandwiches, muffins, soft drinks, hamburgers, even eggs and some fruits are just *bigger* than they used to be. And, not surprisingly, the average American eats about 600 calories a day more than forty years ago.

So how do you eat less, when there's so much food around? You can read labels, measure portions, and use one of the many sites and apps available for keeping track of your caloric intake (www.myfitnesspal.com, www.sparkpeople. com, www.fitday.com, and www.calorieking.com are particularly user-friendly). Especially when starting out, many people find the careful recording of calories that these sites enable helpful.

But you can also eat less without counting calories. Using just your hand, you can estimate recommended portion sizes for various foods:

1 thumb tip = 1 teaspoon of peanut butter, butter, or sugar

 1 finger = 1 oz. of cheese

 1 fist = 1 cup cereal, pasta, vegetables

 1 handful = 1 oz. of nuts, seeds

 1 palm – 3 oz. of meat, fish, or poultry

You probably won't have to rely on this system forever. Just as we've gotten used to oversized portions — when's the last time you saw a fist-sized serving of pasta? — we can get used to thinking of smaller portions as "normal."

Other ways to reduce calories include: switching to smaller plates, bowls, glasses, and cups at home; serving food pre-plated rather than bringing platters to the table; buying single servings of treats (think: ice cream cone instead of half-gallon); packing up leftovers for future meals immediately after eating; and eliminating sweetened drinks altogether.

Mom was right when she told you "breakfast is the

most important meal": studies show that people who eat breakfast, especially if it contains a protein such as milk, cheese, yogurt, peanut butter, or eggs, are much less likely to binge later in the day.

In restaurants, order an appetizer portion instead of a main course, ask the server to take the bread basket away and to bag up half of your meal before you start eating, and look for menu items that are broiled rather than fried, or dressed with olive oil (or not dressed at all) rather than with cream, cheese, or butter. Request a salad, fruit, or extra vegetable to substitute for French fries or other caloric side dishes; order fruit or sorbet for dessert, or share a rich dessert and just have a forkful.

Also, whether you're eating at home or out, *slow down and pay attention*. In one study, women who were asked to take their time and set their forks down between bites ate 10% less than women who ate more quickly—without trying to reduce their intake. Several studies have shown that eating while watching TV causes people to eat more and that eating while driving, in addition to making people eat more, is as dangerous as talking on a cell phone while behind the wheel!

You'll be pleasantly surprised that these little adjustments, which add up to major caloric savings, are relatively painless. Cornell psychologist and expert on eating behavior Brian Wansink calls these small changes the "mindless margin"—calories you would have consumed by eating the last few spoons of rice in the pot, the mediocre mac and cheese that came with the chicken, or that whole piece of chocolate cake that you didn't even really want, and won't miss.

2. Make Healthier Choices

As I mentioned, calories aren't the only consideration. To maintain a healthy body, you need to eat a varied and balanced diet that includes 10-35% of its calories from proteins, 45-65% from carbohydrates, and 20-35% from fats, approximately 30 grams of fiber, plus vitamins and minerals. Within these categories, some choices are healthier than others. For example, monounsaturated fats like olive oil and polyunsaturated fats like vegetable oil are healthier than saturated (animal) fats like lard and butter; beans, tofu, fish and other lean proteins are healthier than red and cured meats; whole grains are healthier than refined white flour products; and the fiber, calcium, vitamins, and other nutrients found naturally in food are preferable to those packaged in supplements.

Here's a more detailed summary of healthy food choices:

Instead of these:	Use these:
Butter, solid margarine, or lard	Olive oil, canola oil, or margarine without trans fats
Cream-based sauces	Tomato-based sauces
Whole eggs	Egg whites or egg substitute

Salt for seasoning	Herbs and spices
Canned vegetables	Fresh or frozen vegetables
Corn flakes, Special K, or other refined-grain cereal	Cheerios, Wheaties, or other whole-grain cereal
Cream of Wheat	Oatmeal (steel-cut oats are best) or other whole-grain hot cereal
White rice	Brown rice or other cooked whole grain
White pasta	Whole-wheat pasta
White bread	Whole-grain bread
Full-fat dairy foods	Skim or low-fat dairy foods
Processed meats	Fish, chicken, beans, nuts
Fatty cuts of meat, such as prime rib	Leaner cuts, such as tenderloin (occasionally)
Smoked, cured, salted, or canned meat or fish	Fresh or frozen meat or fish, without added salt
Sugared soda or juice	Water, or juice mixed with sparkling water
Ice cream	Yogurt with fruit

French fries	Roasted vegetables and potatoes
Candy	Fresh or dried fruit
Chips	Nuts, raisins, popcorn without butter (try olive or canola oil), raw vegetables
Snack crackers	Whole-grain crackers without trans fats
Dips high in saturated fats	Hummus, peanut butter, or seasoned low-fat yogurt
Baked goods containing butter or trans fats	Foods baked with healthy fats
Cookies	Graham crackers or oatmeal cookies with fruit
Super-size restaurant entrées	Small- or medium-size entrées
Fried foods	Grilled, broiled, steamed, poached, or roasted foods

Adapted from Eat, Drink, and Be Healthy: The Harvard Medical School Guide to Healthy Eating by Walter Willett, M.D., (Simon & Schuster and Harvard Medical School, 2005).

In 1992, in an attempt to make healthy eating recommendations easier to follow, the U.S. Department of Agriculture designed the food pyramid. Foods at the wider parts of the pyramid, like fruits, vegetables, and whole grains, were to be eaten more often, and foods at the narrow top, like sweets and alcohol, rarely. But many found this diagram confusing. In one funny cartoon, a person who's clearly not losing weight with the pyramid exclaims: "Oh! I was reading it upside DOWN!"

In 2011, the USDA switched to a plate diagram, which makes a lot more sense. Who, after all, carries a pyramid to the buffet table? Several organizations have come up with their own version of the healthy plate. Here's one from Harvard Medical School and the Harvard School of Public Health:

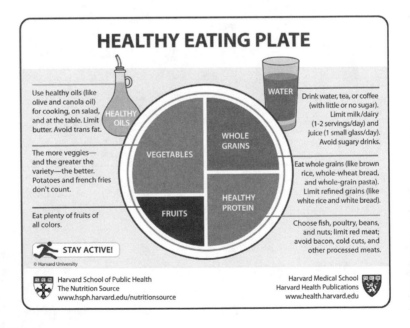

HEALTHY EATING PLATE

Use healthy oils (like olive and canola oil) for cooking, on salad, and at the table. Limit butter. Avoid trans fat.

HEALTHY OILS

WATER

Drink water, tea, or coffee (with little or no sugar). Limit milk/dairy (1-2 servings/day) and juice (1 small glass/day). Avoid sugary drinks.

The more veggies— and the greater the variety—the better. Potatoes and french fries don't count.

VEGETABLES

WHOLE GRAINS

Eat whole grains (like brown rice, whole-wheat bread, and whole-grain pasta). Limit refined grains (like white rice and white bread).

Eat plenty of fruits of all colors.

FRUITS

HEALTHY PROTEIN

Choose fish, poultry, beans, and nuts; limit red meat; avoid bacon, cold cuts, and other processed meats.

STAY ACTIVE!

© Harvard University

Harvard School of Public Health
The Nutrition Source
www.hsph.harvard.edu/nutritionsource

Harvard Medical School
Harvard Health Publications
www.health.harvard.edu

I find the Healthy Eating Plate a useful image to keep in mind, whether you're eating at home or out. Your plate may not be perfect every time, but loading up on vegetables, looking for brown rice instead of white, ordering fresh fruit for dessert, and sticking with water rather than soda, are changes that, added up, make a big difference to your health and waistline.

3. Eat Less Prepared and Processed Food

In general, food that is less processed and, especially, prepared at home— fruits and vegetables; fish, meats and legumes; seeds and nuts; milk, yogurt, and naturally-aged cheeses; whole grains—are healthier than processed and packaged food. Additionally, when you cook at home, rather than buying take-out or eating in a restaurant, you have much greater control over portion size, and avoid the added salt, fat, sugar, and preservatives that pre-made food so often contains— not to mention the money you save and the many pleasures of enjoying a home cooked meal, plus leftovers!

Though many factors have contributed to the rise in obesity and weight-related disease in the past few years, I would vote our increased intake of processed and pre-made foods #1. Currently, cookies, chips, processed meat and cheese, and sugary sodas and energy drinks make up an astonishing 35% of the calories Americans consume. I've seen many women lose weight and even get off blood pressure medication and insulin simply by giving up these unhealthy foods.

As you start eating less processed and more whole foods, you may find yourself wondering whether organic (grown without pesticides) fruits, vegetables, and grains and hormone-free dairy, eggs, and meats are healthier than their convention-ally produced counterparts. Certainly hormones and pesti-cides aren't beneficial, and can be harmful, so it would be best to avoid them when you can. Fortunately, the price of organic, locally sourced, and/or hormone-free foods has been coming down, and these foods are now often available in regular gro-cery stores and discount chains, as well as at the farmers' mar-kets that have sprung up in most towns and all major cities.

When, because of cost or availability, you can't buy all or-ganic produce, keep in mind that some conventionally grown fruits and vegetables tend to retain more pesticides than others. The so-called "Dirty Dozen" are the twelve kinds of produce you either want to buy organically grown, or wash extra-carefully before eating if you don't buy organic. Then there's the "Clean Fifteen," those types of produce where it is less important to buy organic.

"Dirty Dozen" (In other words, try to buy these organic)
- Celery
- Peaches
- Strawberries
- Apples

- Blueberries
- Nectarines
- Sweet Bell Peppers
- Spinach
- Kale/Collard Greens
- Cherries
- Potatoes
- Grapes (Imported)

"Clean 15" (Lowest in pesticides, probably don't need to buy organic)
- Onions
- Avocadoes
- Sweet Corn (Frozen)
- Pineapples
- Mango
- Sweet Peas (Frozen)
- Asparagus
- Kiwi Fruit
- Cabbage
- Eggplant
- Cantaloupe (Domestic)
- Watermelon
- Grapefruit
- Sweet Potatoes
- Honeydew Melon

Reference: Environmental Working Group

While we're on the subject of processed food, what about artificial sweeteners? Don't they help you lose weight? In fact, a 2008 study done by researchers at Purdue University showed that laboratory rats fed artificially sweetened food gained more weight than rats fed food sweetened with sugar. At least one study suggests that people who drink one or more diet sodas a day are also more likely to gain weight. The reasons for these surprising findings aren't entirely understood; changes in metabolism and increased desire for sweets created by artificial sweeteners have both been considered. But one thing seems clear: many people use sweeteners like aspartame (Equal) and sucralose (Splenda) as a way of justifying unhealthy food choices. How often have you ordered a cheeseburger or two slices of pepperoni pizza… with a diet soda? You see this same "logic" at work in coffee shops where people often ask for a skim latte or cappuccino… with whipped cream on top!

Just as an experiment, try avoiding artificial sweeteners. Use a teaspoon of sugar, honey, or maple syrup here and there if you enjoy a little extra sweetness in your drink or on cereal or fruit. (If you have diabetes, discuss this with your doctor or dietician, first.) I bet you won't gain any weight, and you may find a small taste of "the real thing" much more satisfying than several packets of the fake stuff.

A word about supplements: they are greatly overused. The biggest nutritional problem we face as a society is excess, not deficiency, though poverty and hunger are still present at alarming rates. The evidence in support of most nutritional supplements is either poor or evolving. For women over fifty who eat a healthy and balanced diet who wish to take supplements, good daily choices would be: a multivitamin (*not* with iron), 1200-1500 mg of calcium, 1000 IU vitamin D, and 1000-3000 mg omega fish oil (or flax seeds or oil, for vegans).

4. Be Prepared

Yes, it's the Boy Scouts' motto and it should be yours, too. Quick quiz: At the end of a hard day, would you rather have a bowl of homemade soup, a fresh salad, a whole grain roll, a bowl of berries and a glass of red wine... or take-out pizza or Chinese food? At three in the afternoon, when your energy flags, does half a turkey sandwich, some hummus and crackers, or some dried fruit and nuts sound good... or would you be happier with stale, leftover Halloween candy? Which breakfast would fuel you better for an important morning meeting: oatmeal, fruit, and yogurt eaten at home or at your desk... or a doughnut eaten in your car?

No question, sometimes we do crave junk food. Most of the time, though, given the choice, we actually find the healthy stuff more appealing. But so often we don't give ourselves the choice because we don't shop for ingredients and prepare meals and snacks in advance, or carry food with us when we're out of the house. Then what happens? We get hungry or our blood sugar levels drop—at least every 2-4 hours—and we reach for whatever's available. Would you

take a child on a three-hour outing without bringing a nourishing snack along? Would you invite a friend over for dinner
and forget to shop and cook for the meal? Why not provide
for yourself at least as well as you provide for others?

From years of dieting, you may have gotten accustomed
to the idea that weight loss = deprivation. In fact, with a little
preparation, your healthy eating plan will feel like the opposite of deprivation: you'll always have plenty of attractive and
delicious food available.

Here are a few simple strategies for staying prepared:

Stock your fridge and pantry

Diet books often advise you to ban all fattening foods
from your kitchen. It's true that if having boxes of cookies in
your cupboard makes it difficult for you to avoid eating too
many cookies, it's best not to keep them around. But you
also don't want to have one of those homes that contain
nothing edible other than diet soda, diet margarine, and diet
bread, either. Few things make people more anxious — or
more likely to overeat at the first opportunity — than a scar-
city of food. So replace an abundance of unhealthy food with
an abundance of healthy food. Here's a list of staples to keep
stocked — add your own favorites:

Fruits and vegetables: They're all great but the tastiest and
most nutritious are the most deeply colored ones: carrots,
red peppers, beets, dark greens, blueberries, cantaloupe, etc.

Wash, peel and cut produce before putting it in the fridge so that it's easy for you and your family to grab a healthy snack or cooking ingredient. Keep an assortment of fruits and vegetables in the freezer, too. Dried fruits are a good dessert, sweet snack, or cereal or salad topping—but use in small amounts since they're high in calories.

Whole grains: Read labels carefully. "Whole wheat" often means *some* whole wheat with a lot of white flour. Look for 100% whole grain breads, English muffins, rolls, tortillas, pita, cereals, and pasta. Also try brown rice, bulgur, barley, and quinoa for variety.

Proteins: Low fat and non-fat milk, soy milk, yogurt, and cheeses; canned and dried beans, tofu, canned tuna, salmon, and sardines; chicken breasts, ground turkey; veggie burgers; hummus; unsweetened nut butters; nuts (almonds and walnuts are especially healthy).

Fats: Olive oil and canola oil are the healthiest of the oils and good to have on hand for cooking, sautéing, and baking. Avocados and olives are a satisfying source of vegetable fat—but, like oils, high in calories. Flax seeds can be added to yogurt, smoothies, cereals, and salads for some extra omega 3 (the "good" fat also found in salmon and other cold water fish).

Extras: Salsas, pickles, relishes, and mustards are salty, but used in small amounts can really perk up foods, as can hot sauce, herbs, spices, and a variety of vinegars (balsamic, sherry, and champagne are great). Intensely flavorful fruit sorbets and dark chocolate (70% cacao and higher is best) are excellent to have on hand because just a little will scratch the itch for something sweet.

"Default Dishes" and "Little Black Dresses"

Keeping all these good foods in the house is one thing, and eating them is another. If you come home tired and hungry to raw broccoli and frozen chicken breasts you won't eat well…unless you have a plan.

One excellent plan is to have a few "default" dishes — those no-fail, easy-to-make meals you really love to eat. Perhaps these are healthy updates of recipes you've enjoyed for years, or those you've pulled from cookbooks, magazines, or the Internet. Ideally, these are dishes that can either be prepared on very short order, or ones that you can make over the weekend and then re-heat through the week. Many homemade soups and stews, in fact, taste better when they sit in the fridge for a day or more.

A good, basic repertoire to start with would be: a vegetable or bean soup; a chicken or lean meat casserole or potted dish; a vegetarian pasta sauce; a vegetarian or lean meat chili. If you aren't a confident cook, look up recipes for these dishes on the Internet and experiment with the ones that use healthy ingredients and are labeled "easy." Gradually, you'll have mastered a few that will become your "default" or go to recipes. I almost always have, in my refrigerator, a lentil and brown rice stew, a pot of chicken or vegetable soup, or some homemade marinara sauce — all very simple to make (I'm *not* a great cook) and dishes I'm always happy to have when I get home.

In addition to those "default" recipes, I'd like to introduce you to the concept of "little black dress" dishes. You know how every woman is supposed to have a basic "LBD" she can dress up or down for any occasion? (A man in my wellness group asked if he could think, instead, of khaki pants and a blue blazer!) Well, translate that idea to food. Here are some "LBDs" you can "accessorize" to make an infinite variety of healthy meals and snacks in *less than 10 minutes*:

Rainbow salad: In the fridge, layered between paper towels in a salad spinner (I learned this trick from my mother-in-law — it keeps veggies fresh for days!) keep salad greens, sliced peppers, shredded red cabbage, chopped herbs, leftover cooked vegetables, etc. Top a portion of this colorful salad with beans, hardboiled eggs, leftover fish or meat or whole grains (great for those restaurant doggie bag contents), nuts, seeds, jarred peppers, pickles, and artichokes. Splash on some olive oil and vinegar or lemon juice and you have a very satisfying meal, with lots of flavor and crunch.

Stir fry: In olive or peanut oil with a little sesame oil and soy sauce, sauté sliced chicken breasts or firm tofu with veggies from your rainbow stash plus chopped fresh ginger, scallions, snow peas, and bean sprouts. Add a few chopped peanuts or canned water chestnuts.

The Big Burrito: Stuff a whole wheat tortilla with beans, leftover chicken or tofu, veggies, salsa, a little cheese, brown rice. Microwave for a minute or two.

The Little Dipper: Put some yogurt, nut butter, or hummus in a bowl. Dip apple slices, carrot sticks, or whole grain crackers or pretzels.

Trail Mix: Put whole grain cereal in a bowl or small bag with a few nuts, raisins or other dried fruit, and dark chocolate chips.

Oatmeal, Your Way: Microwave 1/2-cup rolled oats with 1 cup water plus chopped apple, banana, raisins, dates, or other fresh or dried fruit topped with a dash of cinnamon or allspice. Top with skim milk or yogurt plus walnuts, almonds, or pecans and, if you like, a few drops of real maple syrup or honey.

Omelet for One: Beat eggs or egg whites and cook in a pan greased with a little olive oil. Add raw or leftover cooked veggies, a sprinkle of grated cheese, salsa. Serve with whole grain toast, or rolled in a tortilla, or cold… on a rainbow salad!

Smoothies to Order: Put a handful of ice cubes, a cup of milk, soy or almond milk, kefir, or yogurt, a banana, and a handful of any kind of fruit (if frozen, skip the ice), plus protein powder and/or flax seeds if you like. Blend.

Topped Potatoes: Keep baked white and sweet potatoes in the fridge. Split, soften the insides with a fork, and microwave with leftover veggies, beans, a little shredded cheese. Top with Greek yogurt, chives, black olives, and salsa.

Personal pizza: Top pre-made whole wheat pizza dough with homemade or jarred tomato sauce, a little shredded cheese, turkey or chicken sausage, peppers, onions, spinach or any other vegetable. Bake according to directions on the dough package.

Get creative. Invent your own "LBD"s... and do send me the recipe!

5. Don't Forget the Treats

Holidays, vacations, anniversaries, birthdays, and other special occasions are some of the most joyful and memorable times of our lives. Any weight loss plan that requires you to pass up croissants in Paris, champagne on New Year's, or your favorite Thanksgiving stuffing, is not one you can stick to — nor should you! The trick is to be choosy about your splurges. They should be the very best versions of foods you really love. If you adore that Thanksgiving stuffing, but feel less enthusiastic about the candied sweet potatoes, then skip the potatoes—don't eat them just because you're "already blowing your diet" with the stuffing. Day to day, if you enjoy dessert, keep it simple. Stick to fruit with a little sorbet or yogurt; or a square of dark chocolate. Save the special treats for special occasions. As a dietician colleague of mine likes to say: "You should enjoy your holidays, but 'Wednesday' isn't a holiday."

Remember that calories do count, even when you eat healthy food. You may find you need to use an online calorie counter or keep a written journal, read labels, and measure portions for a while, or on and off—or even forever, if that works best for you. Your stomach is also a good gauge of when you've had enough. Stopping when you're full, and putting away food for later when you're hungry again, is the best and most natural form of "portion control." But it takes some practice—and many of us are out of practice. You may have grown up feeling guilty about "wasting" food (as if stuffing yourself to the point of discomfort were *not* wasting it) or hearing, depending on your age, about the starving children in Europe, Asia, or Africa. Also, if you're a chronic dieter, you may not feel very confident that the potatoes or cookies that you're gorging on will be available later if you don't polish them off now—because you're so used to starting a new diet that forbids them.

It may seem to go against the way you've always thought about food and weight loss, but keeping your refrigerator, cupboards, lunchbox, and office desk drawer full of healthy and appetizing food, and deciding for yourself when, how much, and what to eat rather than punishing yourself with diets and deprivation, will make you feel calm, well cared for… and less likely to overeat.

Emotional Eating

There's a cartoon that always brings nods of recognition when I show it to my patients: a woman who's spooning ice cream directly from the pint container explains to her concerned-looking husband: "I'm not eating. I'm self-medicating."

The truth is, many of us use food in an attempt to make ourselves feel better when we're sad, anxious, angry, or just plain bored. This is called "emotional eating"—eating that's driven by uncomfortable emotions rather than hunger. A good way to know if you're eating for emotional reasons is to ask yourself where in your body you feel the desire to reach for food. If your stomach feels empty and rumbling, you are likely hungry. But if the sensation you feel when you just *have* to eat something is located more in your upper chest and throat, you are more likely eating to drown out an emotion.

Your choice of foods also gives a clue as to whether your eating is emotional. When you're really hungry, you feel most satisfied by proteins and fat, plus some carbohydrates to refuel the glycogen stores in your muscles (especially if you've been exercising). When you're eating to soothe psychological distress, you reach mostly for sweets and carbs (plus fat and salt), which act directly on the "feel good" centers of the brain. Think about it: what woman has a fight with her spouse or receives an audit notice from the IRS and then goes searching frantically for grilled chicken and greens sautéed in olive oil to cheer herself up?

The truth is, emotional eating works pretty well in the short run — that's why we do it. You do feel better after gobbling a chocolate bar or a bag of chips, for a few minutes. But there are several problems with emotional eating as a coping mechanism. For one thing, it makes you gain weight. Even a very brief episode of emotional eating, in which you're likely to wolf down highly caloric food very quickly, can add hundreds of calories to your daily intake. Second, these episodes often leave you feeling ill and lethargic. That's because if you're not eating to satisfy hunger, you don't have a natural stopping point.

As author and philosopher Sam Keen once noted: "You can never get enough of what you didn't want in the first place." So you keep eating until you run out of food, or you feel too sick to eat another bite — whichever comes first. Finally, and most importantly, stuffing yourself with food does nothing to address the reasons you felt uncomfortable in the first place. So you're likely to get uncomfortable again and again — and react to that discomfort the only way you know: overeating. Plus, overeating often leads to self-blaming, self-punishing thoughts ("I'm so fat!" "I need to go on a diet right away!") which causes even *more* distress, which leads you, inevitably, right back to the cookie jar.

How to get off this merry-go-round? Resolving never to go on a restrictive diet again helps. Threatening yourself with diets really fuels overeating. How many times, after all, have you gone on a "farewell to food" binge right before starting a new diet?

As I mentioned, eating breakfast decreases the likelihood of a binge in the mid-afternoon and after-dinner hours (the most popular times for overeating). I find that women who binge later in the day skip breakfast—because they're still stuffed from the previous night's bingeing! A way to break this cycle is to start eating breakfast regularly, even if that feels unnatural at first. In fact, I'd recommend to anyone trying to lose weight that they "front load" their day's food intake: eating two small breakfasts about 2-3 hours apart, and two light lunches, also 2-3 hours apart, then a light dinner. You'll be amazed at how this routine increases metabolism and cuts that late-in-the-day desire to snack.

The best remedy for emotional eating, however, is to understand and learn to better manage the emotions that lead to it. Trying to control emotional eating instead of dealing with the emotions that cause it is like trying to resist shivering rather than putting a sweater on. It just doesn't make sense.

So what, exactly, do you do with all those unpleasant emotions other than smother them with food? Many diet books suggest all sorts of tactics to distract you from your desire to eat: call a friend, take a bubble bath, etc. These work sometimes—though taking a bubble bath on the street in front of the bakery is tricky!—but I think it's much better to learn a few simple stress management techniques that allow you to calm yourself down without food. You can find many of these techniques in *Chicken Soup for the Soul: Say Goodbye to Stress*, but here are just a few:

- *Wait it out.* Feelings, including uncomfortable ones, tend to be fleeting. Often, if you delay even five or ten minutes, the desire to grab for food passes.

- *Talk it out.* With yourself, or with someone else, try to identify why you feel the need to binge. Are you lonely? Tired? Worried? Is there something that might relieve the problem more directly and effectively than ice cream?

- *Learn to relax.* Close your eyes. Breathe deeply and slowly. Drop your shoulders and un-tense your facial muscles. Even after a few seconds, your blood pressure and heart rate fall, the stress chemicals your body releases when your brain perceives a threat become less active, the urge to eat dissipates.

- *Become more stress-resistant.* Satisfying relationships, meaningful work, hobbies, and community activities, and spiritual fulfillment can all make you less likely to experience those panicky moments that drive emotional eating. Regular exercise, good nutrition, meditation, yoga, tai chi, qi gong, and other relaxation practices have also been shown to reduce anxiety, depression, and psychological distress in general.

Sometimes an inability to manage emotions without over-eating signals a mental health problem, such as anxiety disorder, depression, or post-traumatic stress disorder. If you engage in emotional eating frequently, and find it very difficult to stop, you should consult your doctor. A referral to a therapist or treatment with medication may be helpful.

Severe and frequent gorging may be a sign of an eating disorder. Though eating disorders are often associated with adolescents, even older women may have or develop binge eating disorder (a condition in which very large volumes of food are consumed several times a week) or bulimia (bingeing accompanied by attempts to "purge" the extra calories through self-induced vomiting, use of diuretics or laxatives, or compulsive exercising). If you've experienced any of these behaviors you should also consult your doctor.

The Tiny Waist of the Fifties

She looked like June Cleaver except for her red hair. Like many young mothers in the fifties, mine often did housework in what she called a "housedress." It was nothing like the slouchy sweats I wear today to tackle the toilet bowl, the kitchen floor, and the cobwebs in the corners.

The housedresses our mothers wore then were unique. They were cotton and had to be ironed. They buttoned down the front to about six inches below the waist or nearly to the hem. The waistline of that dress still amazes me after all these years. Mom's waist could not have been more than twenty-two inches. The dress always had a belt that defined her tiny waistline.

That housedress, with its tiny belt-covered waist, represents an era when people didn't discuss or worry about weight control. It was something that happened due to lifestyle. Diet programs and books were much less prevalent.

Most of my adult life, I fought to keep my weight under control. It was a struggle at which I had varying degrees of success. I tried fad diets as well as healthy diets. The struggle occupied too much of my time and thought, almost to the point of obsession.

About three years ago, the image of my mom's belted

housedress began to flit across my mind frequently enough that I deemed it important. I decided to evaluate her lifestyle compared to mine. Surely there was something about how her generation lived that kept most of them trim even into their later years.

Here is what I found:

- We never ate more than one thin pork chop each. When Mom opened a can of vegetables, it was shared by four of us. Our hamburgers were probably about a sixth of a pound. Weekday breakfasts were a piece of toast, milk, and juice. Yet, I never remember passing out from hunger. Conclusion: If we eat smaller portions, we will survive until the next meal.

- We ate a wide variety of fruits and vegetables. Living in an agricultural community, we had access to fresh produce, which Mom canned. Although we had meat at most meals, produce dominated our plates. We always had some type of starch with our meals. Conclusion: Starch is not bad. Meat is not bad. The idea is to use them as additions to our meals rather than the mainstay.

- We ate food close to its source. We did not have packaged food until I was in high school. About that time, the infamous frozen potpie arrived.

It was totally disgusting, so we seldom ate it. Conclusion: There's something about real food that promotes good health.

- Neither of my parents ever obsessed about food. If we had homemade ice cream, we all enjoyed it. I suspect Mom's bowl was smaller than Dad's, but she never mentioned the fact. We all enjoyed the ice cream guilt-free. I think my mom's idea was that if she could get enough veggies into us during the meal, there wouldn't be a lot of room for dessert. Besides, most of our desserts came from the fruit bowl. Conclusion: No food is bad. And, it may be that spending too much time analyzing one's diet causes problems.

- Mom and Dad did all their own work. Mom did the shopping, cleaning, laundry, cooking, sewing, and childcare. Dad did the yard and repair work. They raised chickens and put them in the freezer to enjoy through the year. Together, they painted and papered walls, waxed floors, and cleaned rugs. Conclusion: There was no need for a gym membership when there was so much to do at home.

- Television and computers didn't dominate our lives. Even after we bought a TV, we chose to be active. Although we weren't jogging or working out on a piece of machinery, we were moving most of the time. Even our winter taffy pulls burned more calories than sitting in front of a screen. Conclusion: An active lifestyle is conducive to trim waists and good health.

- We ate supper at six o'clock and had nothing else to eat until breakfast. That gave us about a twelve-hour fast each night. Conclusion: Bodies do well not having a continual inflow of food.

After I looked at how a family of the fifties lived, it was apparent that our twenty-first-century lifestyle was responsible for the differences in our waistlines. I decided to make some changes

I knew any modifications needed to be gradual so I could fully embrace them. Drastic changes usually end in failure.

I set up these guidelines, knowing it would take time to totally adopt them:

- Decrease portion sizes drastically. Picture the one-fourth-can serving size of my youth.
- Plan for my plate to be two-thirds plant-based food, light on white starches.
- Quit talking and thinking about food and diets.
- Increase the amount of work I do in the house

and yard. Include regular gym-type exercise because I use work-saving devices not available fifty years ago.

- Decrease screen time.
- Eat supper early and then fast until breakfast.

Has it worked? It has been three years. During that time, I have very gradually lost fifteen pounds. That is not the "fifteen pounds in two weeks" many fad diets advertise. But slow is okay, because I know I am changing.

I changed how I think about food. I know that I will not fall over if I eat a light meal. It's okay to leave food on my plate. I learned that a meal heavy on meat makes me feel sluggish, so I look for ways to get more vegetables on my plate. I eat my larger meal at noon and try to have a light supper early.

I changed how I feel about exercise. It is now like the air I breathe—necessary for my wellbeing, rather than something I force on myself. I do some weight training and yoga. I walk outside if the weather is nice, or I watch the news while I'm on the treadmill. I have a shelf for my computer in front of the treadmill, allowing me to watch inspiring or educational videos.

What is in my future? I may never totally adhere to my guidelines. I sometimes eat too much. There are times when I eat late. I don't think about food and diets as much as I once did, but here I am writing about them now.

However, I don't believe I will ever again have an issue

with weight. I expect to slowly lose a few more pounds until I am where I should be. I doubt I will wear house-dresses with belted waists even if they do come back in style. It is enough to be strong and healthy, and to have more pleasant things on my mind than the number of calories in a food or whether or not it is "on my diet."

— Carole A. Bell —

The Closet Witch

A sense of dread washed over me when my husband suggested a date night. We hadn't been out together as a couple for months. His invite in past years would have evoked joy. Instead, my insides cringed from knowing I would have to face my clothes closet witch, the wicked monster who silently taunted me.

Even now I remember the nasty questions I imagined emanating from my closet. "What size are you this week? Will those black dress pants still fit? When are you going to lose weight?"

I had attended my daughter's wedding in a full-panty girdle so that I could fit into a dress purchased six months earlier. That was a wake-up call. I began obsessing about my weight gain. Then, within a year of the wedding, the big "M" happened. Yes, and menopause in all its hormonal glory ushered in the birth of the closet witch.

I work from home, so pajama loungewear was my typical dress du jour. It's hardly the type of clothing someone wears to accentuate a shapely figure, and conveniently for me, it hid the mounting pounds. Some people have comfort foods; I had comfort clothes and plenty of them. I found myself staying home more often. The process of finding casual or dressy clothes that fit was a daunting task and staying home meant avoiding the closet.

As my body had grown, so had my closet. There was a

"skinny clothes" section, a "post-skinny clothes" section, and a "fat clothes" section. At some point, to keep my sanity and marriage intact, I moved the skinny clothes to the attic. My weight obsession was driving my husband crazy. He was tired of hearing me complain that I didn't fit into anything. When I officially graduated into the closet's fat clothes section, I became depressed and defeated.

For most of my life, I had been thin. I could down a bag of chips, a chocolate candy bar and can of soda without adding an ounce. In my late thirties and early forties I worked out at a gym five days a week. I was fit and proud of it. When others mentioned weight gain issues, I was clueless and insensitive to their struggles. It's funny how things come full circle. Now I was in my fifties facing weight issues that many family, friends and co-workers had faced for a lifetime. I felt ashamed that I had been less sympathetic to them.

I tried fad diets and quick weight loss programs. Usually these were prompted by an upcoming trip or vacation requiring swim attire. I would lose weight on these diets, but within months I was right back to my mid-life status quo weight. And every regained pound was like quicksand. I was being pulled under by the weight (no pun intended) of knowing I had no long-term plan for maintaining my weight loss and making a lifestyle change.

Then it happened. One morning I stepped on the scale and realized if I didn't do something to lose weight, I would eventually have serious health issues. And my self-esteem could plummet into a black hole from which it might never return. So began my weight loss journey.

The following Saturday my husband clicked on a cooking channel before heading outside to mow the lawn. Over the sound of the humming lawnmower, the television blared in the background. I walked over to turn off the TV but became engaged with the Hungry Girl cooking episode showcasing basic recipes. I was engrossed in the demonstrations of simple healthy recipes geared for weight loss. The recipes seemed so easy and effortless.

I was not someone who enjoyed cooking and I hardly ever did it. But, something about this cooking show captivated me. I had a glimmer of hope that maybe, just maybe, I could cook to lose weight. And that's precisely what I did.

Call it divine inspiration, or an epiphany. Whatever happened on that Saturday morning changed my life. Knowing I would be leaving for a trip to Chile and Argentina in three weeks motivated me even more. This type of business trip with my husband's peers usually included poolside lounging in swimsuits. I visualized that picture and it wasn't pretty. Following the cooking show episode, I jumped online and ordered three Hungry Girl cookbooks. Upon their arrival, I devoured the books like they were snack foods. I composed a grocery list and planned out weekly meals for my weight loss mission. I started eating five small meals a day and was diligent about portions. I limited myself to 1,200 calories per day and included veggies, low-fat meats, carbohydrates and even desserts. Soon I realized the secret was in keeping the fat intake low and using low-fat, no-fat ingredients whenever possible.

To stay motivated, I began making lunches for my daughter. Even now she stops by every morning en route to work to pick up her plated meal. Yes, "plated." I discovered that creatively plating your meal helps you eat slower and consume less. To date, my daughter has lost twelve pounds and continues to enjoy her Blimpy Girl lunches (what I've dubbed my new plated meals). I photograph my plated meals and post them as "Diary of a Blimpy Girl" episodes on my Facebook page to inspire others.

Within a five-month period, I was thirty pounds thinner and still holding eight months later. Date night with my husband is now exciting. In fact, I can't wait to open the closet door. That closet witch has turned into the closet fairy godmother.

~ Denise Marks ~

The Power of Four

Decades ago, my friends warned me this would happen. As I consumed a seemingly endless stream of chocolate milkshakes, strawberry sundaes and banana splits, they'd shake their heads and say, "It's all gonna catch up with you someday." Turns out, they were right.

I'm not sure when I crossed the line from beanpole to beanbag; I only know that one day I was driving and felt an obstruction between my lower back and the driver's seat. Horrified, I realized that the obstruction was me—a roll of fat like a mountain bike tire wedged between the car seat and myself. Yikes!

When I got home, I took a good hard look at my undies-clad self in the mirror. No denying I was a muddle through the middle. More dismaying, though, was that even my legs—specifically my thighs, which I'd assumed would stay toned forever from a lifetime of exercise—were getting, gasp, chunky. How—and when—had this happened? I was eating the same as always (including a dessert every night) and was exercising as much as ever (daily). It just didn't seem to be working anymore. "It," I realized, was my metabolism. Maybe it wasn't on an all-out sit-down strike, but it definitely was on a work slowdown.

I might have caught on sooner if I'd bothered to weigh myself regularly, but I'd always been so thin I never saw the need to "obsess" about my weight. Meanwhile, the pounds were sneaking on, and my body's equilibrium was getting more and more out of whack. The same amount of food plus the same amount of exercise no longer resulted in the same number of pounds. It was obvious that if I wanted to shed some pounds, I'd have to exercise more or eat less.

Cutting out or simply cutting down on ice cream probably would do the trick all by itself. But over the years, I'd given up smoking, drinking and, for the most part, gossiping. Ice cream was my only remaining guilty pleasure. I chose to exercise more.

I already was exercising every day—at the very least, a walk around my neighborhood, which is a good mile. Yoga, swimming, gardening, exercising my horse—one of these "extras" was added to my daily walk more often than not. But a mile walk and an extra activity apparently weren't cutting it anymore. I needed a more disciplined approach. So I devised an exercise point system similar to the food point systems used by dieters.

The system works like this: An easy mile, which takes me roughly twenty minutes, is worth 1 point. All other exercise is assigned a point value relative to that mile walk. A half-mile swim, for instance, is 1 point; a mile swim is 2 points. Gardening for half an hour is worth 1 point. Shoveling the snow can be 1 or 2 points, depending on snow depth and heaviness. An hour aerobics class is 2 points. A half-hour yoga video is 1 point. Mowing the lawn with the power mower is 1 point. Even housework counts—vacuuming or mopping floors for half an hour is worth 1 point.

Through trial and error, I discovered that if I want to eat ice cream and lose weight at the same time, I must earn 4 points a day. The points can be amassed in any combination and at any time of day or night. For instance, I could take a two-mile walk in the morning, mow the lawn in the afternoon, and do a half-hour yoga video before bed. Four points. Or I could exercise my horse for half an hour in the morning, walk the dog around the circle in the afternoon, and take a two-mile walk in the evening. Four points. If I do something exotic that's not on my points menu—someone invites me canoeing, for example—I estimate the number of points based on how much energy I expended compared with a mile walk.

"Cheaters" are partial points that I don't keep track of—parking my car across the lot from the grocery store, taking the stairs instead of an elevator, occasionally carrying hand weights on a walk, etc. The cheaters add up and are insurance against those days when time simply doesn't allow me to reach 4 points. I try to keep those days to a minimum, and have had very few of them.

I do give myself Sundays off, which is a big physical and psychological boost. If I'm beat on a Thursday and it's late and I still need a point, I tell myself "Sunday's coming" and muster the energy for one last walk around the circle or a stretch-and-flex video before bed. Even though Sunday is a free day, I can exercise if I want to and take a walk if the weather's glorious or do some gardening if the weeds are calling. The point is I don't have to.

This system works for me. I'm losing weight—albeit slowly—and keeping it off. I never feel that I'm in an exercise rut, and I like the fact that necessary activities—mowing the lawn or mopping the floors—count toward my points. Another plus is that this system covers all three components of physical fitness—strength, cardio and flexibility. Best of all, I never feel deprived!

Four points a day might seem like a lot to pay for the luxury of eating ice cream, but it's worth it to me. If I want to drop my point requirement to 2 or 3, I can always cut out or cut down on the ice cream. That probably won't be happening anytime soon, though. I just stocked up on Cherry Garcia.

— Kristine McGovern —

An Apple a Day

I never had a weight problem in my younger years. In college, when my friends and I bemoaned our "Freshman Fifteen," I simply gave up dessert and the pounds melted away like ice cream on a July afternoon. In my thirties, I added an hour of aerobic exercise a few times a week and managed to stay trim and fit. Even when I advanced into my forties and gained a permanent five pounds, I felt great and still looked good in a swimsuit.

But then came the big 5-0.

Turning fifty flipped a switch in my body. Within a month, five new pounds established themselves around my middle and wouldn't leave, no matter how much I exercised. Half a year later, those five pounds had turned to ten, and on the cold January day I celebrated my fifty-first birthday, I weighed fifteen pounds more than I had the year before.

Then came the day I couldn't zip a pair of pants that had hung perfectly on my hips a year earlier. Something had to give. I embarked on a diet that included nothing but salad and water. Ugh! I was hungry all the time and felt too tired to exercise. The diet lasted three days, but I continued my exercise: walking two miles a day, several times each week.

Not long after that, a television program caught my attention. The topic was eating habits and how to control hunger. A high-fiber diet makes you feel full. Apples are a great source of fiber and relatively low in calories. Eat one as you prepare dinner, and you'll be able to control your portions more effectively.

Why not? I thought. It makes sense—I'll give it a shot.

The next day I added apples to my grocery list. I ate one just before lunch and another while preparing dinner: a salad bright with carrots, yellow peppers, green spinach, and fat-free feta cheese alongside a new, low-fat Greek chicken recipe I had found in a magazine. I traded my usual glass of wine with dinner for a glass of Perrier. The chicken was delicious, and I was full after one serving. The apple trick was working. Day One of the new me.

My low-fat diet and exercise routine continued, but I didn't see much change when I hopped on the scale each morning. Those pounds were as stubborn as the proverbial mule. I ate an apple with a serving of fat-free yogurt for breakfast and tried not to think about it.

I started walking three miles instead of two and drinking an extra glass of water. My body was not going to win this argument.

Twelve days later, the scale gave in and declared me a winner. I was three pounds lighter when I stepped into the shower that morning. Ridding myself of the extra pounds was taking longer than when I was in my twenties and thirties, but by golly, I was losing weight.

Three more pounds disappeared by the end of February, a glacial pace compared to my younger days. But I was determined to win, determined to lose the weight, determined to get back in those pants I still couldn't zip.

When I went for my annual physical a few weeks later, I stood on the digital scale in the doctor's office and watched in horror as the ten pounds my scale said I had lost registered as only six.

"That can't be right!" I said, wondering how I could pack on four pounds in a few short hours.

The nurse looked at me and smiled. "Does your scale say something different?"

"It must be the wool pants and sweater," I mumbled, stepping off the scale. I wanted to kick it.

I asked my doctor why it was so hard to lose the weight.

"Your metabolism slows down as you age," she said. "Do you exercise?"

"I walk three miles, four times a week."

"That's good. Keep it up. Do any weights?"

I didn't, so she suggested adding some hand weights to strengthen my upper body.

"What about your eating habits?"

I told her about the apple diet.

"It can't hurt," she said. "A woman your age needs extra fiber to stay regular."

Great. Add insult to injury.

I bought the hand weights and another bag of apples on my drive home.

"What's for dinner?" my husband asked when he got home from work that evening.

"Chicken. Any recipe requests?"

"I liked that Greek chicken you made a few weeks ago."

So I made his new favorite dish, eating an apple as I cooked.

The next morning, I added hand weights to my exercise routine. I had to take two ibuprofen that night to battle muscle soreness, but by the end of the week the pain was gone and I had increased the weight repetitions from ten to twenty. Four weeks later, I saw a difference in my arms. The flab was diminishing as muscles developed.

Although I've had a few setbacks, an apple—or three—a day is one of the best secrets to my dieting success. Eating an apple before each meal makes me feel full, which makes portion control a lot easier. And the more I exercise, the better my mood. I really like those little endorphins running around inside my head.

I can zip that troublesome pair of pants now. But best of all, I wore a sleeveless, size-eight dress to my college reunion this past spring.

I found my solution to the problem of the "Fifty-something Fifteen" and it all started with a bag of apples.

— Ruth Jones —

Healthy from the Inside Out

I stepped on the bathroom scale. It groaned, and then revealed that I had gained a significant amount of weight during my painful, drawn-out divorce. At age fifty, I knew that excess weight could create serious health issues. It was time to take action.

Throughout my life I tried fad diets, and with youth on my side I was able to manage my weight successfully. I found it easy to shed the weight I'd gained during my two pregnancies and if I gained weight between Thanksgiving and New Year's, it came off easily with some attention to diet and a little extra exercise.

However, once I hit menopause the weight didn't come off as quickly or as easily as it had in the past. It seemed that if I so much as looked at chocolate cake it would show up on my hips! I realized that if I wanted to win the battle of my bulge I would have to take an entirely different approach to weight loss. I had to make lifestyle changes.

One day, while perusing the health and fitness section of the local bookstore, I came across a book touting the benefits of eating raw.

I began to read about the benefits of eating fresh fruits, raw vegetables, nuts, seeds, and juicing versus eating processed foods, high fructose corn syrup, sugar, and white flour. I was intrigued. I purchased the book and my education began.

I learned that cooking vegetables depletes the vitamin content and can reduce enzymes necessary for efficient digestion. Eating raw vegetables combats diseases such as diabetes and cancer—both diseases prevalent in my family history. Raw vegetables provide an excellent source of fiber, resulting in feeling fuller, longer. As a result, the urge to snack diminishes. Fruit contains a good amount of water resulting in hydration and provides an excellent source of vitamins. The natural sugar found in fruit gives us a boost to get through the mid-afternoon blahs.

After reading the book from cover to cover, coming to terms with the poor food choices I made in the past, and forgiving myself for my ignorance regarding said choices, I was ready mentally and emotionally to move from a sugar-rich and white flour-rich diet to a diet rich in raw foods. I was ready to commit to hard work and discipline so I could reclaim my good health.

Initially, moving to a sugar-free diet was tough. I experienced withdrawal symptoms: headache, diarrhea, nausea, lethargy. Despite all this, I knew my body would benefit and that kept me motivated. I sought support from a friend who was familiar with eating raw and her encouragement helped immensely.

After eating raw for about two weeks I noticed that my skin began to look younger and took on a softer tone. My mind was sharper. I began to sleep soundly without waking in the wee hours for no apparent reason. My heartburn began to dissipate; the antacids I regularly chewed to dispel the discomfort remain untouched. Mood swings disappeared, as did the bloating I had experienced in my fingers and ankles. Not only did I feel great, I looked great, too. For the first time in years I felt healthy from the inside out. An added benefit? Within the first four weeks I lost sixteen pounds and I was ecstatic!

After four weeks, I added exercise to my regimen. I began walking around the outside of the building in which I worked, a distance of half a mile, twice daily during my fifteen-minute breaks. The sunshine provided me with vitamin D. The fresh air gave me a natural high. During periods of inclement weather I'd walk in the mall after work or use a low-impact glider that I purchased at a yard sale. I even got a headset for my telephone so I could talk with friends and family while exercising!

When I reached a weight loss plateau I was not concerned because I knew that my body was adjusting to the new foods, exercise, and vitamins I'd introduced. But when that plateau continued for three weeks I became frustrated. I called my friend for advice.

"Just keep exercising and watch what you eat. Eventually your body will respond," she told me.

Two weeks after our conversation I was still at the same weight. Again, I called her for advice. We talked at length regarding what I ate, when I ate, how much I ate and how much I was exercising.

"Increase your water intake," she recommended. "If you add a little bit of fresh lemon juice or lime juice to the water that might make it easier to drink. It will take some time but you'll definitely benefit from the additional water."

Following her advice, I began to increase my water intake. I drank water rather than coffee during my morning commute. I replaced my mid-morning coffee at my desk with water and included an additional eight ounces on my evening commute home. Drinking additional water became part of my routine and the benefits showed—my joints no longer ached and my skin looked less wrinkled. Best of all, when I stepped on the scale two weeks later I had lost nearly four additional pounds!

I have since continued to lose weight as I have made healthy choices—replacing white flour products with wheat flour, replacing beef with poultry, and by reading product labels to identify unhealthy ingredients. I have maintained my exercise program.

Everyone's life is different. For this reason, I asked a lot of questions to find what would work best for me, would fit into my schedule and allow me to integrate wellness into my personal routine in an enjoyable way. The methods that had worked for me when I was younger didn't work once I turned fifty. However, by making a few lifestyle changes I have improved my overall health. This has been the path to my success—a path I will continue to walk for the rest of my life.

~ Elisa Yager ~

Mom, Eat Your Vegetables

I am excited about dinner tonight. I'm going to make vegan chili and it is so easy! I'll pour a can of corn, a can of black beans, a can of red beans, a can of white beans, and a double-sized can of diced tomatoes in a pot, along with potatoes, onions, carrots, peppers, and whatever other fresh vegetables I find in the fridge, season it with salt, pepper, cumin, chili powder, and a little cinnamon, simmer it for an hour and serve it over rice. I'll have enough leftovers for several dinners for two and lots of lunches for me to take to work. It will freeze great. And it's as easy as opening cans.

Other nights, when I'm tired, I toss carrot sticks, halved fingerling potatoes, and onion chunks in a baking pan with olive oil, kosher salt, pepper, and thyme, and roast them at 400 degrees for thirty minutes. The carrots come out tasting as sweet as candy and it is a hearty and filling meal. Even my husband doesn't feel deprived, despite the fact that I have served him only vegetables. And I get leftovers to take to work.

I've been a much bigger fan of vegetables ever since our two younger children "went vegan" last year and my daughter, who is in medical school, showed us the film *Forks Over Knives*, which makes a strong case for the health benefits of a plant-based diet. This doesn't mean that I am going vegan like my children, foregoing all animal products, including milk, eggs, and even honey, but it does mean that I have rediscovered how wonderful fruits and vegetables and whole grains are and how they make fabulous main courses. I eat very little meat, poultry, or fish now and I have significantly cut back on eggs and milk products, substituting soy and almond milk for cow milk.

My husband and I feel better, thinner, and more energetic, and have a lot more fun eating dinner. By focusing on plant-based meals, I am able to make delicious stews or pasta dishes from whatever we have in the house, all in one pot. I always cook extra, so that I can take single servings to work for lunch and also have plenty of leftovers for future dinners. I have even started serving plant-based meals to our friends at our dinner parties and they are very receptive.

Last summer, before my daughter started medical school, she was home enough to spend a lot of time in the kitchen with me. She taught me to use Earth Balance instead of butter, how to use delicious spices like cumin to make vegetable dishes tastier, and how to be creative and flexible when fashioning plant-based meals. This Christmas, she tried to teach me how to make kale, that super leafy green that is so full of protein and nutrients. I had heard of kale but thought it was somewhat mysterious and scary. When I came home from Whole Foods one day proudly bearing what I thought was a big bunch of kale, she informed me that I had actually purchased a large head of romaine lettuce.

My son gave me a vegan cookbook for Christmas and the

kids left my refrigerator filled with things I don't know how to use, such as nutritional yeast and flaxseed meal and wheat germ. I'll figure it all out eventually, but for now, one thing at a time. I finally purchased and made kale the other day. It's funny to think that I was afraid of a giant leafy vegetable!

This whole plant-based eating program happened at just the right time because I have gotten much more serious about eating properly in the last couple of years. I've never had a weight problem, but in my late forties I gained a few pounds. After Christmas one year, I realized I was about to turn fifty and I went on a serious diet, losing a whole size in time for my fiftieth birthday party that April. But then I started my job as the very busy publisher of Chicken Soup for the Soul and the weight came back.

This became a problem two years ago when I was working on our *Chicken Soup for the Soul: Shaping the New You* book with Richard Simmons and I was planning to visit Richard in Beverly Hills and take one of his rigorous exercise classes. This was an emergency! Luckily, the book was very inspirational and I learned several excellent lessons from it that worked for me, including:

1. If you're not hungry enough to eat an apple for a snack, then you don't need a snack.

2. Take the stairs whenever possible, which works well in our office building where we are three floors up from the parking garage.

3. You don't have to eat things that are bad for you just because they taste good. If you already know exactly what that piece of chocolate cake will taste like, why not just imagine the taste but forego the fat and sugar and calories?

4. Decaf coffee or tea is a great substitute for a late-night snack.

5. It helps to have an accountability partner, someone to honestly share your food journal, exercise log, or weigh-ins. And if you can e-mail someone your food journal right after dinner, so that you can't eat anything more that night, that is even better!

Through portion control and exercise, I managed to lose that whole size again and went off to see Richard feeling much better about myself. As we publicized the book, I felt that I needed to be an ambassador for its message, which was a great inducement to maintain at my new weight so that I wouldn't let my company down.

Then my gynecologist told me it was finally time to go off the pill. And guess what! I lost another whole size. I must have been carrying weight from the pill for years without realizing it. That was a really nice surprise and made me feel much friendlier towards the whole concept of menopause!

Then the kids turned vegan, as I mentioned, and my

daughter and I started e-mailing each other a food journal every day. I lost a few more pounds and bought new clothes.

But my accountability partner, my daughter, doesn't want to spend the time on the daily e-mails and I have regained a few of those pounds. I really needed the accountability of disclosing my food choices to her every day.

So you, dear reader, are my new accountability partner. Writing this story for Dr. Koven to include in her book has motivated me to focus more on my exercise program and on my plant-based diet. I find that if I eat a "plant-strong" diet as much as possible, the weight stays off, I feel comfortable in my new clothes, and I feel more energetic. It is a delicious way to stay in shape without counting calories, without going hungry, and without feeling like I'm making a sacrifice. And according to that *Forks Over Knives* movie, it is cutting my risk of cancer and other diseases too!

~ Amy Newmark ~

Voices

I didn't need a Mocha Coconut Frappuccino last Friday night, but I wanted one. A sugary coffee drink wasn't good for me; I knew that. Why would I want extra calories after I'd told my husband and my sister I was trying to lose weight? (Menopause has added a whole new dimension to my life—and my waistline.)

I didn't want the drink because I was hungry. My gut still felt full after supper: broccoli soup, carrot sticks, and half a grilled cheese sandwich made with 100% whole grain bread. A low-calorie meal (except for the cheese) with lots of antioxidants. I racked up at least two vegetable servings for the day with that supper.

No, I wanted a Mocha Coconut Frappuccino because I wanted it. The drink offered me a nice end to an exhausting week. I planned to order the light version with sugar-free syrup and non-fat milk. Plus I had a treat receipt from my husband's coffee purchase earlier in the day. My sweet indulgence would cost me only $2. Just $2 for a little shot of happiness. How could I waste such a bargain?

I had it all worked out in my mind. I wouldn't have to make a special trip, because there was a Starbucks inside the nearest Target. I could redeem the treat receipt after I finished picking up toilet paper and paper towels with no gas wasted.

So I headed to Target, fully determined to reward myself.

Once there, I decided I could walk off some calories in advance if I walked fast. I grabbed a cart and charged down the main aisle, burning rubber the whole way to Paper Goods. Then I wheeled through some other departments to scorch a few extra calories.

Thirty minutes later I returned to the front of the store and paid for my purchases. Then I walked over to Starbucks. The big moment had arrived; there were no customers in line. I laid my receipt on the counter and gave my order to the petite blonde behind the counter.

"Sorry, ma'am. We don't have any sugar-free syrup for that drink. Or any sugar-free syrup for the chocolate drinks. I can use the non-fat milk, but you'll still get all the calories of the regular syrup. Or you can have a light caramel drink or a vanilla light. I have sugar-free syrups for those."

But I didn't want caramel or vanilla. Not that I don't like caramel, but my taste buds had anticipated mocha and coconut. I was ready to ignore my full stomach for something worthy like chocolate, but for vanilla or caramel? No way. You can burn only so much energy shopping for toilet paper.

And that's when it happened: I heard voices. With no warning, all the dieting mantras and "eat wisely" slogans from every television expert and magazine article in my past began racing through my brain.

Think about what your body really needs.

Are you hungry, or are you just thirsty instead?

If you're thirsty, drink a glass of water.

Empty calories add real pounds.

You have to take care of your body.

The risk of a heart attack or stroke increases if you're over fifty.

You'll have to exercise for an hour to make up for this.

Nothing tastes as good as being thin feels.

When the voices in my head stopped, I was still staring at the menu board. The girl was waiting; I needed to make a decision.

"Sorry, I've changed my mind. I don't really want caramel or vanilla, and I can't afford the extra calories for the other drinks. Thanks for your time, but I'm not ordering anything tonight."

I picked up the treat receipt and rolled my cart to the door.

My dad was diagnosed with Type 2 diabetes at age sixty, as was his mother. I'm only five years away from that mark. Friends and relatives my age have already battled serious cancers. If I was diagnosed with cancer next month, I'm not sure whether my body would be ready for the fight.

Like many women my age, I know what I should do when it comes to my health. I've read the articles and watched the health stories about baby boomers on television. I've heard the fitness gurus encouraging me to make wise food choices and get moving. I listen to their advice most of the time, but sometimes I don't want to listen. I want the voices in my head to be quiet.

Last Friday I listened to the voices, and they were right. I didn't need a Frappuccino or a bunch of meaningless calories. I needed a glass of water, and I could get that at home.

~ Donna Savage ~

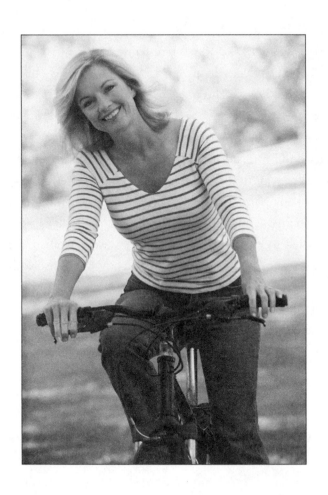

Chapter 5
The Long Run

The Long Run

To Live, Not to Diet

I once had a fascinating conversation with a friend of mine, an observant Jew. She told me that while she found it impossible to stick with a diet, she had no trouble keeping kosher, a special way of shopping for and preparing foods according to Jewish law that requires quite a bit of effort. When I asked her why she thought this was so, she thought a while and then answered: "It's because I *do* a diet…but I *am* kosher."

This is the secret to long-term success with weight loss and fitness: you repeat the same behaviors so often that they become part of your identity. Think about other behaviors you do automatically: do you argue with yourself every day about whether you should brush your teeth, buckle your seatbelt, or wash your clothes? No. You do these things because they make your life healthier and more comfortable, but also because you've done them so many times that it would feel weird *not* to do them. These activities have become part of who you are.

You can feel the same way about healthy eating and exercise. The stories in this book are about people who not only changed their habits—they transformed their lives. The couple who've gone for a walk after dinner every night for decades, the woman who's still doing yoga in her nineties, the woman who cooks vegan dishes with her daughter no longer have to worry about being "on program." That's not to say there aren't days they don't feel like making the effort, but they keep doing it anyway. Woody Allen once said: "Eighty percent of success is showing up." Just keep showing up: to the gym, to the kitchen, to the yoga mat, to the hiking trail.

But what about when your motivation flags? Experimenting with new recipes and new kinds of exercise may help. Taking on fresh challenges, like running a road race or climbing a mountain, may renew your enthusiasm. "Row Strong, Live Strong" and "The Silver Streakers" are both stories of women who kept upping their game. Even a new piece of kitchen equipment or exercise outfit can give you a jumpstart.

Reassessing your motivation periodically is also important. Though disease prevention may be a major benefit of eating healthfully and exercising — and I hope I've convinced you that it is! — studies show that avoiding illness isn't always the most potent motivator for behavior change. I remember a woman in one of my groups who told me she was determined not to get diabetes like her mother, who'd suffered a leg amputation from the disease. I suggested to her that, awful as the prospect of sharing her mom's fate was, it didn't seem to be spurring her to eat differently or to exercise — and she acknowledged this was true.

Two other factors have been shown to be at least as powerful, if not more powerful, than health in helping us sustain a new lifestyle. This first is whether the behaviors we are trying to adopt give us joy in the moment. You know that wonderful feeling you have, maybe at a wedding, around a holiday table, or just finger painting with a child, when you wouldn't want to be anywhere else than where you are just then? If you feel that way while nourishing or moving your body, you will want to keep repeating that experience. You won't need to worry about "will-power." In "Keep It Steady," Monica Morris describes the blissful feeling she experiences routinely in a Jazzercise class, and many contributors to this book recount the feeling of peace and well-being they have simply by eating well and exercising.

The second thing that spurs us on— more and more as we get older —is the desire to leave a positive legacy. Don't you want your children and grandchildren to remember you as vital and energetic, a role model for how to age well? And, whether or not you have children, don't you want to play your small part in turning back the tide of obesity and preventable disease that threatens the health of present and coming generations? The World Health Organization estimates that by the year 2020 two-thirds of all disease will be related to unhealthy lifestyles, especially excess processed food and lack of exercise. Reversing this trend will involve public health measures, changes in farming practices, urban planning, and other large-scale efforts. But it will also require that individuals like you and I, one by one, decide to lead healthier lives.

Back to Exercise

I am grimy. Grimy like floor-of-the-Port-Authority-bus-terminal-after-rush-hour grimy.

I have been lying on the floor of the exercise studio, hoisting myself into push-ups with a five-pound weight on my back. I have been slamming a medicine ball at my exercise partner and catching it as she slams it back at me. I have jumped down from a high step repeatedly, jumped rope, and climbed up and down the bench in a kind of crazy quickstep. And that's just in the first forty-five minutes!

I don't think I have ever sweated more or felt more fatigued. Yet I couldn't be happier. I am back in my exercise class after nine months of absence. I had to stand aside because of a knee injury.

That day on the tennis court when I ran full steam ahead from the baseline to get a drop shot at the net turned out to be the beginning of a bad year. I was one step away from the fuzzy yellow ball and when I stepped forward to connect, it was as if I'd stepped into a hole. There was nothing under me and I went down in a heap, as my knee gave way. As I fell, I heard a snap inside my leg.

Following an X-ray, MRI and an examination by an orthopedist, I was told my anterior cruciate ligament was torn "less than fifty percent" and in those cases surgery is not recommended. A few months of physical therapy, and I'd be good to go. I was as dutiful about rehab as a puppy who anticipates a dog biscuit. I did the exercises at physical therapy. I did them at home. I did them at the gym. Three months later, the doctor gave me the green light, fitted me with a knee brace, and sent me on my way.

I marked my return to physical health by rejoining my women's softball team. In my first at bat, I reached first base on a fielder's choice. With two outs, the first base coach told me to "run hard" as soon as the next batter hit the ball. I did. One step away from second base, and again, my knee collapsed on me.

"Maybe you need surgery," the physical therapist said the next morning when I called to share my woe. The doctor said the same thing. So I went for another opinion, to a doctor who only worked on knees. One month later I scheduled the operation.

When I awoke from the surgery, which repaired my torn meniscus and replaced (with a cadaver's ligament) my ACL, I didn't feel as bad as I feared I would. But let's just say this is major surgery, and recovering is not easy. I couldn't drive for three weeks (the hazards of a right knee repair). I watched a lot of TV (favoring *The View* and, I admit it, some game shows).

For someone who has always been active, being debilitated was eye opening. How much I wanted to just go out and run. How much I wished to be able to simply walk my dog. It made me realize how often I catch up with a friend by taking a walk with her. I couldn't even think about tennis, but found that I was missing the women whom I'd meet on the court each week. Mixing friendship and exercise has long been my secret for staying motivated. And most of all, I missed the exercise class that left me feeling so grimy.

With much determination and a lot of hard work, I got the post-surgical okay to return to full activity. I'm much more confident now—now that nine months have passed since the surgery, and I can feel the difference in my new knee.

So here I am, feeling my lungs about to explode in my chest, and noticing the exercise endorphins lifting my mood. I'm happy. Happy to return, happy to recover, and happy to know that though my body betrayed me once, I can now get back to the business of taking care of it—all over again.

~ Andrea Atkins ~

Life on Foot

I t began over thirty years ago when my husband and I realized that we were never able to finish a sentence, let alone a paragraph, in a household in which three spirited daughters were coming of age. We realized at about the same time that we'd forgotten the simple pleasure of putting one foot in front of the other and taking a walk. And not on a treadmill at some gym, but outside in what my grandmother used to call the "fresh, clean air."

The inspired idea: We would take a walk every evening after dinner, and discover not just why we'd decided to travel the road of life together, but also get to really know our town. Hadn't we moved to this place, after all, because it was such a pretty, Norman Rockwellian-kind of place with a true Main Street?

So one June night, it began. Two weary people who would have gladly collapsed on the family room couch after dinner, we forced ourselves to open that kitchen door and hit the tree-lined streets. Initially, we hated it.

Huffing and puffing—a testament to our disgraceful lack of fitness—we marked out a route: up a nearby street, down another, left at the next, and so on. My husband, the quantitative sort, did the math: we'd cover 2.3 miles.

We almost didn't make it on the second night. That family room sofa looked mighty inviting, and we would happily have surrendered to it. But one of our kids issued the ultimate challenge: "So are you guys quitting already?"

Nancy didn't know that she was shaming us into decades of almost-daily walking.

Off we marched, slamming the kitchen door behind us. No way were our kids going to have such lethal ammunition to use against us.

When the original route got terminally familiar, we devised two others. When those, too, became ho-hum, we looked for new roads to conquer, at least figuratively. Moorestown, New Jersey, our hometown, we discovered, was bigger and more interesting than we'd realized. And it was a perfect town to conquer on foot.

Over the years, new patterns evolved. As our daughters grew up and left home, we sometimes took to walking later. The neighborhoods we'd explored by dusk looked different after the 11 o'clock news. Often, we were the only souls out and about by the light of the moon, meandering past the local convenience store or the firehouse.

Many nights, we had our best conversations on those streets. We also argued, laughed, walked off anger and celebrated simple joys like the changing of the window décor at the local gift store and real estate office, or the delicious smell of the grass on East Oak Avenue after a summer rain.

On daytime walks, we would stop to buy a few groceries at the little old supermarket where the checkers may not know your name, but they surely know your face. Unlike the big, modern mega-supermarket bruisers all around it, this little place was a reminder of the old corner grocery, and we celebrated it every time we dashed in for a quart of milk or a dozen eggs on one of our daily rambles.

The kids left, and still we walked. Middle age was upon us, and with it the usual renunciations: tricky backs, insomnia, an urgent need for stronger glasses. But somehow, a walk always helped.

Somewhere in our late fifties, we changed our routine. We increased our walking distances incrementally, just to test ourselves, and discovered that with just that little effort, waistbands were looser and our annual blood work was coming back with better numbers.

We also were finding that the loneliness of that famous empty nest was alleviated if we both knew that come nightfall, we could commune. Corny as it sounds, we also drew closer at this "just you and me, kid" stage.

"Save it for our walk," I'd urge my husband when he was about to share an idea, a snippet from his day, or even just a joke. That postponing somehow made the notion of zipping up heavy jackets as the January winds howled a bit less ominous. My guy had a great anecdote for me—and I had a big idea for him.

I could never count the number of vacations planned on our walks, the family problems solved, the home renovations imagined and largely discarded. Ditto for the world crises resolved, the budgets debated, the books analyzed.

Almost more than our physical health, our nocturnal walks did wonders for our emotional health. If one of us was down, the other could sense it and try to help. So many times, one of us needed a shoulder, or gave one.

Not to brag, or tempt the fates, but I wear a smaller size now than I did in my twenties. I love slipping into size-eight pants—but more than that, I love the feeling of robust good health that I enjoy.

Walking—not strolling, mind you, but walking briskly and regularly—has lowered our weight and raised our self-esteem.

Over our long years of walking, the simple gifts of our town's streets have given us a sense of connection to place. I suppose urban dwellers would find it utterly weird that we actually care about how this or that stranger's fence or patio or garden is coming along, but to us, it's second nature.

Besides, we have a reputation to maintain. We've become known in our tiny universe for our year-round walks, and occasionally, when we've been on vacation, neighbors will ask in alarm whether we're all right. And the ultimate compliment? It came recently from a woman at the cleaners dropping off her dry cleaning as I was picking mine up. She stared at me for a long moment, then said, "Oh, I recognize you. You're the street-walker!"

I took it as a high compliment.

~ Sally Schwartz Friedman ~

92 Years Fit

I am ninety-two years old, oddly free of aches or pains. I tip the scales at the same weight—127—I did when I married my husband Sieg sixty-eight years ago. But in the decades between, my weight has changed hugely—once too much, once too little—and I have a figure problem that still makes me work daily to keep it under control.

The problem began in 1952 when I was thirty-two. Living in a small town in upstate New York, we already had two daughters not yet in kindergarten, and were expecting twins.

On the sizzling August day our boys arrived, I checked into the hospital at 172, a gain of forty-five pounds during a full-term pregnancy. I stuck out so far in front I could balance a shampoo bottle atop my bulge. Our twins' combined birth weight—just under fourteen pounds—subtracted a welcome load but I was left waddling around with extra fat and a sagging abdomen that persisted.

Of course some of my weight began to drop since, except for nighttime sleeping, I had to be on my feet almost non-stop. As a stay-at-home mom of four kids under five and a half, I cooked, cleaned, washed, ironed (in those pre-wash 'n wear days), ran errands, and cared for our lively brood. Summers, I tended a garden to help put food on our table.

Necessity made us follow a sensible diet leaning toward plenty of fruits and vegetables with limited amounts of fish and chicken. On my husband's slim elementary school teaching salary, our budget seldom allowed costly items like steak or sweets.

Despite this natural trimming down, and later years when we did a lot of walking, bicycling, swimming, my middle stubbornly kept its post-babies bulge.

Fast forward to 1980, the year I turned sixty. Our children were grown, busy with their lives. By this time my husband and I both had good teaching jobs, with a semester's paid leave ahead when we could do anything we wanted. We thought it would be great to hunt for a very different experience abroad.

This was the time when Hmong refugees, trying to escape war in their native Laos, were pouring across the Mekong River into temporary camps in northern Thailand. Volunteers were needed to teach English. We applied, and were accepted.

On a snow-packed January day, we flew from Iowa, where we lived, to the West Coast. After a trans-Pacific flight, and a long wearying bus trip north of Bangkok, we settled to work in a hot, dry, primitive camp called Ban Vinai. It proved a fascinating, rich plunge into an exotic other world. But the challenge had just begun. We had no facilities to cook for ourselves. There was no grocery in camp, just one open-air fruit and bread market and one less-than-appetizing restaurant open only at lunchtime. Squadrons of flies buzzed both places. All volunteers had been given two warnings if we wanted to avoid amoebic dysentery, a very nasty tropical disease—NEVER buy raw food from that market; eat only cooked meals in the restaurant.

We did our best to shop by bus once a week at a tiny village twenty miles away, but little food was available there. Literally starving, both of us lost a fifth of our body weight in just nine weeks. The day I felt so weak I could no longer stand up to teach and instead crouched on my heels before class, Sieg said, "We've got to cut and run before they carry us out of here in a wheelbarrow."

We hated to walk out on our responsibilities, but back to the U.S. we flew. During a brief airport stop in San Francisco, we each indulged in a huge raw vegetable salad and a double chocolate milkshake—which left me faintly nauseated.

At home, my bathroom scale said I weighed 100 pounds. There was now so little padding on my spine I couldn't bear to lie down in the bathtub. It took months of slow restrained eating to regain our normal weight and strength. During that time we made an interesting discovery: our stomachs had shrunk so much that very small portions satisfied us without hunger pangs. But I was dismayed that despite my extreme weight loss, despite the passage of twenty-eight years since the twins' birth, I still had pudgy, saggy-baggy skin amidships.

For several reasons including cost, I wasn't willing to put myself under the knife for a tummy tuck. Was there anything else that might possibly help this annoying condition?

A newspaper notice caught my frustrated eye. Our local hospital was offering a beginning hatha yoga course. Hmm, I thought. If I froze into one of their pretzel positions, or some day in class fell from a tree pose and broke a limb, a hospital would have first aid handy. I enrolled.

Nothing horrible happened. Quite the opposite. The course not only helped firm my abdomen. It brought me a marked improvement in flexibility, and new techniques of deep breathing that eased me later through two cataract operations. Best of all, it gave me a lasting sense of body control from my middle. It made me feel as if I were standing taller, able to move with a bit more grace. That first yoga course turned me into a strong supporter of formal exercise classes, especially past fifty.

Now I live with my husband in an independent apartment in a retirement complex that offers residents a wide range of free fitness programs.

This has let me keep up yoga, try a year of t'ai chi and four months of Zumba Gold (these are mostly Latin-American dance steps, done individually, and tailored to senior participants). I'm also currently taking two Pilates classes a week—one on floor mats, one in the water. Both work on core strength and balance, but I've found "planks"—those extended body stretches—are far easier in water than on land.

Fortunate genes, an always-moderate diet (our five grandchildren laugh because we habitually get eight servings from one doughnut), and regular exercise combine to keep my weight steady, joints flexible, my middle firmed. This means I can still wear favorite old clothes from twenty years ago.

Since I have no knee or back problems, I plant and tend long areas of flower gardens outside our door every spring and summer in comfort and pleasure—so far.

Although too polite to say "at your age," younger friends

often ask me, "How on earth do you manage to stay in such good shape?"

"There's no secret," I tell them. "It's simple. D for Diet and E for Exercise adds up to D-E-LIGHT."

— Lois Muehl —

Saying Goodbye, for Now

I've shared with you what I've learned, as a doctor and as a woman, about losing weight and getting fit over fifty. Now I'll share one more thing: a confession. When I began writing this book I had not taken consistently the advice I'd been giving to my patients. (This is very common, alas, among doctors!) But reading these stories, and laying out all the evidence of how eating well and exercising improves women's health and lives, inspired me. I now walk or jog almost every day, I lift weights twice a week, I take a yoga class regularly, I keep my fridge stocked with "default dishes" and ingredients for "little black dresses"—and I've never felt better in my life. Those extra pounds came off but, much more important, I now have the energy to do all I want to do, including helping women over fifty lose weight and get fit!

That's my story. Are you ready to write the next, healthier and happier, chapter of yours?

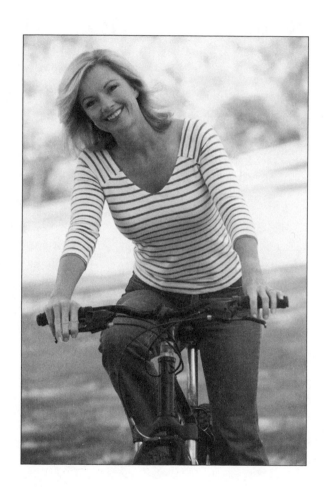

Meet Our Contributors
About the Author
Acknowledgments

Meet Our Contributors

Gloria Ashby is a writer, speaker, and teacher. She publishes "Glimpses of God," a church newsletter column, and writes inspirational stories about God encounters. Living in Texas with her husband Jim, Gloria enjoys reading and digging in her butterfly garden. E-mail her at gloria.ashby7@gmail.com or read her blog at http://gloriaashby.wordpress.com.

Andrea Atkins is a writer whose work has appeared in many national magazines including *Woman's Day* and *More*. This is her second contribution to the *Chicken Soup for the Soul* series. She is married to David I Iessekiel and has two daughters.

Carole A. Bell is a licensed professional counselor. Her ministry is helping families become what God wants them to be. She writes, speaks, and consults about parenting issues. Since 1999, she has written a weekly Christian parenting column for the *Plainview Daily Herald*. Read her blog at www.ParentingfromtheSource.com.

Carol Bryant is a full-time travel agent, part-time nurse, freelance writer and occasional model living in Colorado. She travels the world as often as possible and she is a wife, mother of two grown daughters and a mediocre tennis player.

Terri Elders, LCSW, lives near Colville, WA, with two dogs and three cats. Her stories have been published widely, including in a dozen *Chicken Soup for the Soul* books. She's a public member of the Washington State Medical Quality Assurance Commission. Terri blogs at http://atouchoftarragon.blogspot.com. E-mail her at telders@hotmail.com.

Beth Fortune is an award-winning freelance writer who strives to encourage and motivate others through writing and speaking. She and her husband are empty nesters living in Simpsonville, SC. She enjoys reading, gardening and, of course, indoor rowing. E-mail her at fortunebeth@ymail.com.

An honors graduate of the University of Pennsylvania, **Sally Friedman** has been writing personal essays for over four decades. Her work has appeared in *The New York Times*, *Ladies' Home Journal*, *Family Circle* and *Brides*. She is a mother of three and grandmother of seven. E-mail her at pinegander@aol.com.

Valerie Frost is an office manager for the Facilities Department at Horizon Christian Fellowship, in San Diego, CA. Valerie and her husband, Terry, are the parents of three grown children. They have nine amazing grandchildren, and two turbo-charged Jack Russell Terriers named Daphne and Rocket. E-mail Valerie at tvfrost@aol.com.

Joan Hetzler has written plays, short stories, poetry chapbooks, and is working on a memoir. For eight years, she hosted and produced *The Writers Show*, a radio program for writers in Chattanooga, TN. She also freelances as a technical and communications writer.

Ruth Jones lives in Cookeville, TN, with her husband Terry and a very fat cat named Annabel.

Kelley Knepper is a graduate of Huntington University, Huntington, IN, with a degree in Business Administration and Management. She does accounting work for a local insurance firm in Lafayette, IN. Kelley's hobbies include scrapbooking, painting, crafting, and writing. She especially loves spending time with her family and friends.

April Knight is an author and artist. She loves cats and believes every cat she has owned has enriched her life. She is currently living in soggy, dreary Seattle where the sun never shines. Learn more at www.cryingwind.com.

Mary Laufer is a freelance writer, substitute teacher, and new grandmother. She recently moved back to Florida to be near her son and his family. Walking continues to be an important part of her life, but instead of looking out for ice, she now watches for rattlesnakes and alligators!

Denise Marks runs a successful online global soap making business. She designs and creates molds for chocolatier and soap manufacturing companies. Blimpygirl.com is an offshoot of Denise's many creative venues. She has a business degree and has published articles in soap making magazines and how-to blogs. E-mail her at infor@blimpygirl.com.

Kristine McGovern is a former newspaper journalist who now edits books and writes plays at her home in Centennial, CO. She enjoys painting, swimming, and riding her horse, and she has no intention of giving up dessert. E-mail her at krmcgovern@msn.com.

Monica Morris lives and writes from her big old farmhouse in rural Illinois. She is wife to Joe, mom to Katy and new mother-in-law to Chris. Monica attended the 2008 Guideposts Writers Workshop and her articles have appeared in *Guideposts* and *Angels on Earth* magazines.

Lois Muehl, retired teacher of English in high school, universities and abroad, began writing prize-winning books for children when her four were small. Now living in Iowa with her husband of sixty-seven years, she continues freelance writing, especially poetry. Her hobbies include reading, crafts, yoga, exercise and gardening.

Amy Newmark is Publisher and Editor-in-Chief of Chicken Soup for the Soul and co-authors many of the books as well. She and her husband have four grown children. You can reach Amy through webmaster@chickensoupforthesoul.com. Follow her on Twitter @amynewmark.

Helen Reeves was a reluctant redhead all her life. A native of New Mexico, she plays piano and is a dedicated tango dancer. She works and lives in Iowa City, but she'll dance anywhere.

Suzanne Ruff is the author of the recently published book, *The Reluctant Donor*, described by critics as a "beautifully written, gut-wrenching memoir" and a finalist in the MIPA Book Awards. www.thereluctantdonor.com. Suzanne is a freelance writer for the *Charlotte Observer Mooresville News*. E-mail her at ruffsuzanne@gmail.com.

Donna Savage is a pastor's wife and teacher who helps women embrace their problems with faith and joy. She plunged into freelance writing as an empty nester and has published hundreds of articles and devotionals. Donna and her husband Hoyt live in Nevada. Contact her at donnasavagelv@cox.net or www.donnasavage.blogspot.com.

Simone Sheindel Shapiro retired from a career in computers to focus on her husband, children and grandchildren, and her passions in life: travel, running and fitness, Spanish, photography, Jewish history, and writing. She helps Pittsburgh senior citizens stay fit with her personal training business, Buff Bubby. E-mail her at BuffBubby@gmail.com.

Marilyn Turk has started the next chapter in her life as a writer after a thirty-two-year sales career. Her works have been published in *Guideposts*, *Clubhouse Jr.*, *The Upper Room* and other

Chicken Soup for the Soul books. She and her husband live in Florida, where they enjoy fishing, golf and tennis.

Lois Wickstrom is a former chemistry teacher who currently acts as Imagenie on YouTube. She writes children's books, including *Nessie and the Living Stone*, *The Reluctant Spy*, and *Grippy and Cormo's Magnet Activities*. She is married to the love of her life, has two children and four grandchildren. E-mail her at reluctantspy@gmail.com.

Elisa Yager is a regular contributor to the *Chicken Soup for the Soul* series. When she's not writing, Elisa can be found doing something involving animals, history, or yard sales. She has a passion for stone houses and hopes to one day own one when her publishing "ship comes in!" E-mail Elisa at author_elisayager@yahoo.com.

About the Author

Suzanne Koven is a physician and writer in Boston. For over twenty years she has practiced primary care internal medicine at Massachusetts General Hospital and served on the faculty of Harvard Medical School. Her clinical interests include weight and stress management, women's health, and mind-body medicine. She writes the monthly column "In Practice" for *The Boston Globe*, where she also regularly contributes essays and reviews. Her weekly blog, "In Practice," appears at boston.com/health. Her work has also been published in *Psychology Today* and elsewhere.

A frequent public speaker, Suzanne has addressed health professionals and lay audiences on diverse topics including menopause, work-life balance, nutrition, exercise, end-of-life care, and—her passion—the role of narrative or storytelling in medicine.

Suzanne was born and raised in New York City. She received her B.A. in English literature from Yale, and her M.D. from Johns Hopkins. She also holds an MFA in nonfiction from Bennington. After completing her medical training at Johns Hopkins Hospital in Baltimore, she moved to the Boston area where she now lives with her husband and—when they're home—three grown children. When she's not writing or taking care of patients, Suzanne loves to read and travel. She tries to practice the healthy lifestyle she preaches, and appreciates that her patients continually remind her how rewarding that endeavor can be.

Please visit Suzanne's website:
www.suzannekovenmd.com

Follow her on Facebook at:
Suzanne Koven MD

Follow her on Twitter:
@SuzanneKovenMD

E-mail her at inpracticemd@gmail.com

~

Acknowledgments

No first-time author could wish for more generous support from mentors, colleagues, patients, friends, and family than I've had. I thank:

- Grace Dane Mazur, novelist, critic, and extraordinary writing teacher, for setting me on the path. Also, Maxine Rodburg, another magnificent writer and teacher, who, when I told her, somewhat sheepishly (at the Harvard Faculty Club), that what I'd really love to write was a realistic and slightly irreverent book about weight for women of a certain age, replied: "I'd read that!"

- Sven Birkerts, Susan Cheever, Dinah Lenney, Phillip Lopate, and Wyatt Mason of the Bennington Writing Seminars, for showing me what it means to be a professional writer.

- Gideon Gil, Thomasine Berg, and Nicole Lamy, my editors at *The Boston Globe*, for helping me stretch my writing wings.

- Suzanne Russell-Curtis R.D. C.D.E., Leah Giunta F.N.P., and Marcy Bergeron A.N.P., my colleagues at

Massachusetts General Hospital's Bulfinch Medical Group Cardiovascular Disease Prevention Program; Ms. Jean Tempel, visionary supporter of the CVD program through Bulfinch Medical Group's Patient Doctor Partnership; and, especially, the patients who've participated in the program, as well as the hundreds of patients over the years who have shared with me their efforts to live healthier lives and my brave "pioneers" in the Women, Weight, and Wellness group. This book got its start in what I learned from you.

- Sarah Schultz and Mary Duffy-Zupkus P.T., M.P.A, who lent me their expertise during many conversations about exercise, fitness, and the psychology of change.

- Julie Silver, MD, Chief Editor of Books at Harvard Health Publications and passionate champion of physician-writers, for giving me the opportunity to write this book, and Natalie Ramm, her assistant at HHP, for unfailingly cheerful and skillful help with the manuscript.

- Amy Newmark, Publisher and Editor-in-Chief at Chicken Soup for the Soul, for being so smart and so open-minded. I'm spoiled for life, editor-wise.

- My true co-authors, the remarkable women who contributed their stories to this book. You made me smile, nod in recognition, and put on my sneakers even when I didn't want to.

- Lastly and mostly, my wonderful husband Carlo, and our three amazing children: Sophie, Tony, and Giancarlo: Your love and laughter make *everything* better.

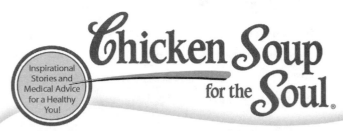

Chicken Soup for the Soul:
Boost Your Brain Power!
978-1-935096-86-3
ebook: 978-1-611592-10-8

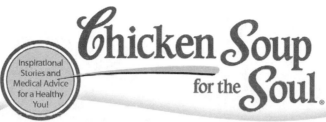

Chicken Soup for the Soul.

Inspirational Stories and Medical Advice for a Healthy You!

by **DR. JULIE SILVER** of
HARVARD MEDICAL SCHOOL

Say Goodbye to Back Pain!

How to Handle Flare-Ups, Injuries, and Everyday Back Health

Terrific tips for flare-ups *and* for chronic back pain.
You'll be back in action sooner than you think!
~ Dr. Howard Ezra Lewine

Chicken Soup for the Soul:
Say Goodbye to Back Pain!
978-1-935096-87-0
ebook: 978-1-611592-08-5

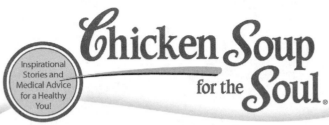

Chicken Soup for the Soul.

Inspirational Stories and Medical Advice for a Healthy You!

by **DR. JEFF BROWN** of
HARVARD MEDICAL SCHOOL
with **LIZ NEPORENT**

Say Goodbye
to
Stress

Manage Your Problems, Big and Small, Every Day

Fantastic advice on how to reduce stress and restore
serenity to your life. Who knew it could be so easy?
~ Dr. Amy Gagliardi

Chicken Soup for the Soul:
Say Goodbye to Stress
978-1-935096-88-7
ebook: 978-1-611592-09-2

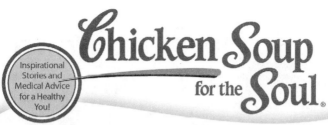

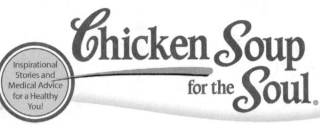

Chicken Soup for the Soul.

Inspirational Stories and Medical Advice for a Healthy You!

by **DR. JULIE SILVER** of **HARVARD MEDICAL SCHOOL**

Hope & Healing for Your Breast Cancer Journey

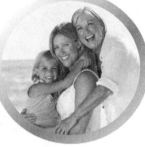

Surviving and Thriving During and After Your Diagnosis and Treatment

Every woman diagnosed with breast cancer deserves excellent emotional and medical support— this book delivers both! ~Dr. Kimberly Allison

Chicken Soup for the Soul:
Hope & Healing for Your Breast Cancer Journey
978-1-935096-94-8
ebook: 978-1-611592-11-5